THE
I · LIKE · MY
BEER
DIET

THE
I · LIKE · MY
BEER
DIET

MARTIN R. LIPP, M.D.

M Evans
Lanham • New York • Boulder • Toronto • Plymouth, UK

Library of Congress Cataloging in Publication Data

Lipp, Martin R., 1940–
I-like-my-beer diet.

Bibliography: p.
Includes index.
1. Reducing diets—Recipes. 2. Beer. 3. Drinking
behavior. I. Title.
RM222.2.L535 1984   613.2′5   84-13561

ISBN 978-1-59077-295-9

M Evans
An imprint of Rowman & Littlefield
4501 Forbes Boulevard, Suite 200
Lanham, Maryland 20706
www.rowman.com

Design by James L. McGuire

Manufactured in the United States of America

Distributed by National Book Network

To
Naty, Michelle, Melissa,
and Sanford

Acknowledgments

Few books reach print without help from others, and certainly this one had its share of assistance from friends and family. For careful reading and criticism, for suggestions and items of beer trivia, I want to thank Sister Deb and Brother Paul, Gusto Charles, Fast Philsie, the Ingerbrewers, Singing Carol, Friend Jeff, Cousin Peter, Wild Willie, and the whole Sack family. Amiable Amy helped with research. Mila did the typing, and Jack and Sammy provided support. Fritz Maytag helped years ago in convincing me not to open a beer store. The United States Brewers Association was generous with information, as were many brewers. To them all, I extend my great appreciation.

Contents

THE
I · LIKE · MY
BEER
DIET

OPENERS

If you didn't like to eat, you wouldn't be reading a diet book—
and if you didn't like to drink, you wouldn't be reading *The
I-Like-My-Beer Diet*. The combination of eating and drinking,
usually such a satisfying component of the flow of days, has
unfortunately added unwanted pounds to your frame; and you
are therefore in the unhappy circumstance of consulting a diet
book, probably not for the first time.

Alas, the days are over when you, as a young savage, could
eat and drink without restraint, every day, every week, every
month of the year. As a consequence, your weight periodically
reaches the point where a mirror becomes an adversary, or
you lack the breath to move your bulk from one place to another at the rate you would prefer to go, or your clothes cease
to fit. The elasticity of your appetite once again has outdis-
tanced the elasticity of your waistband.

If you are like me, you have responded to these grim realities by trying a variety of so-called fad diets or by attempting
some "sensible" changes in life-style in order to bring your
life in concert with what nutritional scientists say is good for
you. Fad diets have unfortunately been the subject of an increasingly bad press of late (more about that later), and living
your life sensibly is not very exciting. Rigid devotion to a nu-
tritionally balanced, scientifically approved dietary regimen
has always seemed to me to be the mark of a dreary mind. I
accept it among my patients, but I don't approve of it among
my friends.

Nutritional science just conceivably may be logically sound, but I too often detect a brittle unsoundness in those people who espouse it. More about that later as well.

The I-Like-My-Beer Diet is a fad diet, like so many before it. I say that without apology. Fad diets have their usefulness, and if this one appeals to you, I trust you will find it very useful indeed. This one is different, however, in two important respects: first, of course, is that you get to drink beer. Not even the Drinking Man's Diet, popular two decades ago, allowed you to do that, largely because it was based on a near-paranoia, of carbohydrates, of which beer has a small amount. The next chapter gives beer its due.

The second unique factor about this diet is the principles on which it is based and the daily diversionary items, one set for each of the twelve days of the diet. We will get to all these in due course.

WHY BEER?

Why beer?

Indeed, why *not*?

Beer is the quintessential American beverage. As a nation, we drink more beer than tea, wine, whiskey, or fruit juice. We produce more beer (twice as much, in fact) than any other nation, and our country has five out of seven of the leading brands of beer in the world.

Beer is a staple in our ordinary diet, and it can profitably be a staple in our reducing diet. The myth that beer is fattening is simply that: a myth. The ordinary 12-ounce container of beer contains 150 calories, less than a comparable volume of apple juice (174) or milk (240) and about the same as an equivalent amount of unsweetened grapefruit juice or half a cup of cooked lima beans (ugh). Even a cup of cottage cheese (172) or three thin slices of bologna (184) make beer look like a diet wonder.

Beer got its diet-busting reputation because a small percentage of its consumers quaff their brews in outlandish amounts. The simple fact is that one gets fat on beer only by drinking it in huge quantities, or—even better—by consuming copious amounts of beer *and* platters full of food as well.

Yet beer has many advantages as a diet component, aside from its modest number of calories. Consider the following:

Beer is filling. Unlike many other foods, and especially unlike many "diet foods," beer helps us to achieve the satisfying sensation of a full belly. All those tiny bubbles, so pleasant to watch as they seek the heights from the bottom of your glass, expand your stomach and turn off disquieting hunger signals. *Beer feeds the mind as well as the body.* Let's face it: very little of the eating we do is the consequence of hunger for food itself. Instead, we often eat out of nervous habit, gluttonously feeding the beast inside. One of the lovely gifts that beer provides us is relief from tension. The alcohol of course plays its pharmacologic role, but the beer lover also has the satisfaction that comes from being with an old friend. Drinking beer soothes all the senses: the eyes respond to the amber invitation; the hand grasps the stein in an action as familiar and reassuring as a handshake; the ears hear the pop of the tab or the bottle top and listen to the liquid gurgling into the glass; and taste and smell tumble over one another with pleasure and stress-reducing sensation.

Beer is the most sensible social beverage. We humans are social beings, and social occasions often push us to consume more food and beverages than we might if left to our own devices. Still, life requires compromises and a human being must make them. The fastest and surest way to lose weight is through fasting, but total self-denial is no fun at all and incompatible with a reasonably sociable existence.

Beer, if you take your time consuming it, allows you to be sociable and to drink alcoholic beverages along with everyone else, but has the dual advantage of having fewer calories and less alcohol per unit volume than any other alcoholic beverage. The result is that you can drink cordially without getting either fat or drunk. A 3-ounce martini or Manhattan, for example, has about the same calorie content as a 12-ounce beer, but disappears much more quickly and packs a much larger alcoholic punch. A standard mixed drink (1½ ounces of bourbon and 8 ounces of cola) has about 250 calories, compared to the 150 in a beer with 50 percent more volume. (Many mixed drinks can be substantially more calorific; and unless you are mixing it yourself, you never know quite what goes into one.)

A standard 6-ounce glass of white wine has about the same number of calories as a beer twice the size and, again, a much greater clout in alcohol content.

Beer is nutritious. Around the turn of the century, beer was routinely advertised not only as the beverage of moderation in alcohol consumption, but also as the most nutritious alcoholic beverage. In addition to a large amount of water and a small amount of alcohol, beer contains substantial numbers of B vitamins (including niacin in significant quantities) and modest amounts of carbohydrates and protein. The calories in whiskey, in contrast, are "empty calories," in that they derive only from alcohol and are useful solely for energy if they are used up quickly—but tend to pickle your tissues if you don't burn them up promptly. It is ironic that beer makers don't advertise the nutritional qualities of their products. It's one of the lasting legacies of Prohibition that they are prevented by law from doing so.

Beer is healthful. Chronic ill effects from alcohol, it is agreed, commonly occur with an average intake of 80 grams (of alcohol) per day. The average beer contains 12 grams per 12-ounce bottle or can, or 24 grams at the level of consumption suggested in this diet. At this level, the alcohol is not only not harmful in the average person, it has a manifestly positive effect on life span and particularly on the cardiovascular system. A number of recent studies published in respected medical journals suggest that moderate drinkers (e.g., those who drink two or three beers a day) have a smaller risk for heart attack than teetotalers or even occasional drinkers. Since heart disease represents one of our major obstacles to a long and healthy life, especially among males, one would do well to ponder these observations at some length.

Beer makes a wonderful evening snack. Meals form much of the structure around which we build our lives. Most diet books emphasize that we do best not to snack, and who can argue? Yet many of us *do* snack, and many of us likewise enjoy a drink to sip in the late evening, while reading or talking or watching TV, before going to bed. Beer is ideal for this purpose. Not only is it filling, as noted before, but it can have wonderful sedative properties for someone whose tension level might otherwise forestall sleep. Most people think it's the alcohol that does it, but that is only partially true. Hops, the principal flavoring agent, is a wonderful and gentle sleep-inducer, so much so that Europeans have in the past stuffed their pillows with dried hops, so that the aromatic essence would help speed them on their dreams. A tasty glass of your favorite brew can do the same for you.

A SIX-PACK OF PRINCIPLES

Before moving on to the diet itself, we can profitably spend some time discussing the reasoning behind the I-Like-My-Beer Diet. Sensible people like to have reasons for embarking upon a new course. It is also true that motivation is the key factor in any diet. It will be easier for you to stick to your diet if you understand what it is about, how it works, and why it makes sense for you personally.

Herewith, then, is a six-pack of principles upon which this diet is based.

CYCLIC DIETS

The alimentary trail attracts more than its share of true believers, people who are convinced that they are absolutely correct and everyone else absolutely wrong. For these food fanatics, nutrition is an essentially moral occupation and every item on your menu can be weighed in ethical terms.

I have no personal objections to people who spout nutritional dogma. I am sure that they are otherwise harmless people. As a physician, however, I find that they are prone to nervous exhaustion—which they usually attribute to food additives and environmental pollutants—and that they are so maddening to live with that their friends and relatives are often driven to seek medical help for nervous stomachs, migraine headaches, and the like. As a last resort, some such friends and relatives have even taken refuge in an excess of drink. How dispiriting it is to live with individuals whose sense of personal worth is based not on who they are and how they behave with their fellow human beings, but rather on regular small platefuls of yogurt, sprouts, and unblanched almonds!

One principal dogma of many nutritionists is that every reducing diet must result in prolonged weight loss in order to be considered desirable and effective. Nothing upsets these folks more than the observation that most people with pudgy tendencies will not stay on diets for very long—and of those who do, few will lose much weight—and of those who manage to lose weight, few will keep that weight off for any length of time. In other words, instead of conforming to scientific dogma dictating how they should behave, human beings seem to prefer to live life "unscientifically": losing weight for a while and then gaining it back again.

Very few people I know are interested in living their lives "sensibly" all the time. Who wants to forfeit for all eternity the pleasures of a truly groaning table? Life for me is at its happiest when I gorged myself on barbecue yesterday; I'm sitting down to second and third helpings of linguini today; and I'm looking forward to cheesecake and brandy later . . . and the promise of other splendid repasts fills my future.

Life, I think, should be lived with a certain negligence, a bemused trust in the generosity of Providence. The vast, hollow spaces inside us are God-given, and how we fill them is a test of our character, creativity, fortitude, and perhaps even heroism. Ultimately, the question of how to eat is the question of how to live, and I prefer to do both with gusto.

There are, however, additional considerations. There is a kind of fat that looks good on a person, a corpulence that basks in candlelit rooms, enhances any dinner table, warms conversation, and pleases friends and loved ones. A certain roundness of demeanor blunts the lean and hungry look, encourages confidence and trust.

Yet as we grow from Mother's little pot-licker to become robust trenchermen and -women in adulthood, our sincere appetites threaten to augment our pleasing roundness into a bulk that is sometimes best described in terms of gross tonnage. The scale becomes a reproach that words cannot equal, but words do crop up, carrying no reassurance. Who among us is comfortable with the label "obese"—or even "fat"?

Each of us, then, is faced with a quandary. If I continue to eat as before and continue to gain, I will split all my clothes and incur a large clothing bill. If I simply cut back a little so as to keep my weight stable, I will continue to feel physically uncomfortable and will simultaneously deprive myself of one of life's greatest pleasures—unrestrained eating. The final alternative is to quickly knock off 5–15 pounds in as painless a manner as possible, then resume my customary eating habits. It is this latter course that many of us have chosen repeatedly, and that is the subject of this book and various other fad diets.

In my judgment, there are only two socially acceptable reasons for dieting: first, in extreme cases, because one's weight presents a clear and immediate threat to one's life or health (and this matter does not fall within the scope of this book); and second, to prepare one's body for the happy prospect of zestful and expansive eating in the future.

There are many of us whose weights go up and down within limits more or less acceptable to ourselves, with the range influenced by social and cultural and personal preferences— and also by the food and festivities that Providence thrusts our way. We are not alone. Binge dieting and binge eating have been part of the cultural fabric since the beginning of recorded time. Where the food supplies have been variable in amount and quality, man has gone through periods of relative abstinence—either out of choice or by force of circumstances—and the conclusion of these fasts or diets have most commonly been celebrated by unrestrained gorging. Most primitive peoples wove periods of restricted eating into their village rituals—and celebrated their conclusion with great feasts. The Cherokee, Choctaw, and Natchez Indians all preceded their harvest feasts with lengthy fasts. The restricted forty-day diet of Lent is traditionally followed by an Easter feast. Many cultures have used some form of dieting or fasting as a preliminary to a marriage or other important ceremony or seasonal festival.

In point of fact, it is extremely difficult to prove that a person's health is adversely affected by a pattern of intermittent periods of weight loss and weight gain in the 5- to 20-pound range. Like so many other things, the notion that short-term use of fad diets is necessarily harmful is itself a fad.

CALORIES IN AND OUT

Diets are, of course, a bore. Since what we really like is unrestrained eating, having to limit one's food intake in any consistent fashion over even a limited period of time is probably not going to be a popular topic. Nonetheless, we need to know exactly what it is we are trying to do—and why and how we are going to do it.

The wonderful truth about diets is that almost all of them work . . . perhaps not for everyone, but for many individuals. The key is simply finding one that you can tolerate, and then following it as closely as possible. Fortunately, this diet has been designed specifically to cater to your tastes and quirks as a beer drinker.

The key ingredient common to all diets is that, in order to lose weight, you must burn up more food than you consume. Some diets—the exercise diets—concentrate on the burning-up part, some focus on the consuming, and some make suggestions about both.

Of those that focus on consuming, all have some system for helping you to keep track of what you put in your mouth.

Some tell you to count calories. Some count calories for you, and tell you to eat a portion of this or that, or give you the same kind of information in "dietary equivalents." Some treat you with a dose of theory about proteins, fats, and carbohydrates—and then dope out a formula of what proportion of each is best for you to lose weight. However they do it, all seek to control what you put in your mouth.

The most commonly used systems are based on calorie restriction, usually by reducing or eliminating the most calorific part of our diet: fats. Many of the popular diets in recent years have also cut back on carbohydrates, emphasizing proteins as the major dietary component. A recent extremely popular example of this low-calorie, high-protein diet is the Scarsdale Diet, but variations on the same theme have been around for decades. Among the many that have followed the same general approach in the past thirty years are Irwin Stillman's *The Doctor's Quick Weight Loss Diet* (1967, written with Samm Baker), Dr. Martin Schiff's *Miracle Weight Loss Guide* (1974), and Dr. Frank Field's *Diet Book* (1977).

These diets have been popular because they work!

The I-Like-My-Beer Diet is also a high-protein, low-fat, low-carbohydrate diet, based on a calorie intake of about 1,000 calories per day. Nutritionists hate diets that follow this pattern—every bit as much as the general public loves them—so you ought to know what the critics have to say.

Q. Some people say that diets of less than 1,200 calories per day are dangerous. How about it?

A. If you have the sort of mind that enjoys quibbling over numbers, we are in the range where some folks recommend caution. *Consumer Guide Rating the Diets*, for example, says: "You should not normally go below 1000 to 1200 calories a day, unless you do so under a doctor's close supervision." At 1,000 calories, our diet sneaks up beyond the recommended supervision range; but if in doubt, consult your own physician. For perspective, you may be reassured to know that a recent review article in the prestigious *Annals of Internal Medicine* concluded that even diets of under 800 calories a day are usually safe for as long as three months, under supervision. If you are in good health to start off with, twelve days on our diet should cause you no problems at all. However, if at any time you feel sick, as opposed to simply cranky and hungry, stop the diet and consult a physician.

Q. Nutritionists say that high-protein diets are unbalanced, and warn that they don't contain enough carbohydrates for normal body function. Is that true?

A. It's certainly true in part. We have purposely attempted to "unbalance" the diet by reducing fats and carbohydrates. However, whether you will therefore not have "normal body function" is subject to debate. Try it yourself and see. If you don't think your body functions normally, then stop. *You* are the person who is the expert on your own body. It is extremely unlikely that a slightly overweight person, otherwise in good health, will have any difficulty with body function in the twelve days outlined in this book. No one recommends that you be on this diet forever.

It is also true that high-protein diets such as the one recommended here must be distinguished from the so-called liquid protein diets that have been associated with some significant health problems. Most liquid protein preparations are commercial blends of predigested proteins sold as a gooey syrup. While beer is a liquid that contains some small amount of protein (albeit more, I have read, than an infant in Biafra gets in a week), the bulk of the protein you will consume in this diet comes from groceries that are a familiar part of everyone's ordinary menu.

Q. Nutritionists say that high-protein, low-carbohydrate diets produce the wrong kind of weight loss, mostly water. Diets of this type tend to produce in the body chemicals called ketones, resulting in a state of ketosis, which results in loss of appetite and fluid loss. Is this true?

A. Of course it's true that ketosis is produced. That is to our benefit because, as the nutritionists point out themselves, ketosis helps to diminish appetite. Ketosis is something that happens to all of us under ordinary circumstances. Whenever you fast for a day, you get ketotic. If you booze it up on a Saturday night, you are likely to be ketotic on Sunday morning. If you run a marathon or participate in any prolonged physical exercise on an empty stomach, figure on ketosis. Ketosis is something you know and have experienced many times before. It becomes a health concern only in someone whose kidneys don't function well, or if the body doesn't get enough fluid to wash the ketones out, or if it lasts too long. If you are in good health, it shouldn't be a problem. If in doubt, check with your doctor. As for the fluid, the I-Like-My-Beer Diet will give you plenty.

Q. Nutritionists say that dieting can bring on attacks of gout or hypoglycemia. Is that true?

A. Yes, *any* diet can aggravate gout in someone who is prone to it. On the other hand, being overweight isn't so great for gout, either. Take your choice. It is also true that dieting tends to lower your blood sugar, and for some people that means weakness, easy fatigability, and even nausea. If so, you have to decide whether it's enough of a problem to prevent you from following the diet. Again, this is a diet intended for healthy people who are simply overweight. Anyone with kidney problems, liver disease, gout, diabetes, or active ulcer disease should forget it—as should any woman who is pregnant. If in doubt, check with your doctor.

BALANCING RISKS

All of which brings us to another important point: that of balancing risks. There is no medication that is without side effects. There is no human activity that is without risk. That can be said of eating, working, and even thinking. It is true for sex and for sleep. If you spent all your adult life hiding from danger between the sheets in the security of your own bed, you would still face hazards: your bones would lose calcium and become very fragile—and think of the living you would lose out on!

You know all these things, of course, yet it is a fact of contemporary existence that I can't offer you the I-Like-My-Beer Diet without a discussion of the potential hazards involved, lest someone misuse the diet, suffer injury, blame it on the diet, and haul me and my publisher into court.

This diet is designed for someone who wants to be able to lose 5–10 pounds over twelve days—and still be able to enjoy a beer or two—or even three—each day. It is not designed for drunks, or for people who want to hide from life in the fantasy of liquid freedom. I have never been enthusiastic about people who drink doggedly, continually to excess, without flair or a sense of time and place. I assume that the average reader already drinks alcoholic beverages to excess, at least intermittently, and that the regimen submitted here represents, if anything, a reduction in alcohol consumption. In any event, food and beverage consumption needn't be discussed as though it were a moral enterprise. The potential hazards of immoderate alcohol consumption are well known and need not be restated here. Beer is the least alcoholic of all conventional alcoholic beverages, and even the small amount of alcohol that it contains is absorbed more slowly than the alcohol from whiskey or wine. Still it is possible to get a significant (and therefore potentially troublesome as well as potentially pleasant) blood alcohol level by drinking a couple of beers—

especially if you do so on an empty stomach, under circumstances where you have been dieting for a couple of days. Therefore, proceed with your usual good sense and an extra measure of caution, especially if contemplating doing any driving.

It is also true that people who consistently and chronically use alcohol as a principal source of food energy frequently encounter alterations in their normal body chemistry. It is extremely unlikely that you will have such problems with a couple of beers a day, but—since your total food consumption is reduced so substantially in proportion to those beers—the prudent beer drinker will take a few precautions.

Alcohol interferes with the absorption of several water-soluble vitamins, especially folic acid (folate), thiamine (B_1), and B_{12}. Because your fat intake will be substantially reduced, your intake of the so-called fat-soluble vitamins will also be reduced, that is, vitamins A, D, and K. Under the circumstances, it makes good sense to take a good multivitamin each morning, making sure that it contains at least the minimum daily requirement of folate, thiamine, B_{12}, A, D, and K.

Actually, as a beer drinker, you ought to know a bit more about thiamine. The humorist I. S. Cobb once said that "the liver has a low visibility, but it is easy to hit." The liver can be thought of as the body's chemical factory. When alcohol screws up the body chemistry, the item that is most likely to be screwed up is thiamine. Physicians routinely give supplementary thiamine to drinkers who have been consuming booze to excess. It's one of those rare scientific opinions that has become so widely accepted that it is established as fact. A number of scientific papers have even been published suggesting that alcoholic beverage producers fortify their products by putting thiamine into the bottle along with the brew. However, unless and until that is done, you can help prevent thiamine deficiency yourself, especially when you have been overdoing it—or even during this diet—by taking supplementary thiamine. If your multivitamin doesn't contain at least 10 milligrams of thiamine, you can buy the thiamine separately at a health food store or pharmacy and take it every morning along with the multivitamin tablet. I usually take 25 milligrams or more of thiamine each morning.

A final comment about risks: I hope you'll find this a handy way to lose several pounds rapidly. As we'll discuss later, this needn't be a one-shot deal: I go on the diet anywhere from two to four times a year, depending upon how creative and generous the various cooks I know have been. However, it is not meant to be used as a continuous dietary regimen. Make certain you return to a normal diet after the twelve days are up.

FEELING FULL

If you too have an appetite that never relaxes, you know that a persistent reality during a diet is simply keeping your ravenous hunger from intruding into every waking moment. There is no ideal solution to this problem. These are only compromises—and some tricks to pacify your insides.

One problem that many of us beer drinkers have is that we often reach for a beer to quench a thirst. Twelve ounces (and 150 calories) disappear in less than a minute and we are ready for our second. It's a great way to live, but a lousy way to diet. Contrary to myth, beer is not the world's best thirst quencher: according to research studies, it ranks a poor seventh behind water, club soda, iced tea, coffee, diet cola, and presweetened Kool-Aid. The trick, then, is to treat the thirst with water, a full 12 ounces, and *then* drink the beer in a comfortable, leisurely fashion, savoring the taste you love so well. In fact, I recommend that you always drink a 12-ounce glass of water before each beer. It's a cinch to do at home, not very difficult at a restaurant, and occasionally a pain in the neck at a bar. Simply tell the barkeep that you want your beer with a water chaser, only you want your water first. Explain about the diet. Give the barkeep a nice tip. Most will understand and cooperate.

Water has a number of advantages. It fills you up, and it slows you down when it comes to fork lifting at the table, as well as hoisting the beer. It combats any tendency toward dehydration, which is a consequence of alcohol consumption—though it must be pointed out that beer is mostly water itself and consequently is the least dehydrating of alcoholic beverages. Water likewise tends to flush waste materials from your body, especially those that are a normal consequence of a reducing diet—the ketones referred to earlier.

While a glass of plain water is aesthetically the most pleasing way for me to dampen a thirst before beer, water also can be consumed in other ways—depending on circumstances and time of the day.

In the morning, at home or at work, a cup of hot tea or coffee (without sugar or cream) is a great way to quiet a complaining stomach. Have as many as you like. If caffeine nerves are a problem, or if your stomach acts up or your heart goes pitty-pat, switch to a decaffeinated brand.

In the afternoon, low-calorie soft drinks can serve the same purpose. Whenever your stomach starts talking to you, one or more of these can do wonders. They are filling, some even have reasonably pleasing tastes, and they have essentially no calories. Drink as many as you can stand. If you are a conscientious objector where artificial sweeteners are concerned, try club soda or mineral water instead.

You can also use water as an ally in another way: by helping to create a full sensation before you start your meal. Simply have a full 12-ounce glass of water either before or during your meal—or substitute coffee, tea, club soda, or diet beverages if you prefer.

There are two complications worth mentioning. First, of

course, is that if your body is adequately hydrated, you won't show the dramatic weight loss in the first few days that occurs with the fluid loss inherent in many high-protein diets. That's all right. You'll still lose the weight you want—albeit more slowly—if you follow the diet conscientiously.

Second, water in the gullet is very much like water in a funnel. You are merely a convenient device for transporting the fluid from the glass to the toilet. Be positive about it: time spent in the bathroom is time spent away from the dining table. Each trip is a distraction from your stomach, and therefore a gift.

DIVERSIONS AND DISTRACTIONS

For many of us, food is the warp and woof of our lives. It forms the fabric that clothes our days. Eating and drinking provide the setting in which we meet friends, form the structure around which we weave our schedules, and are our rewards at the end of the day.

It's not surprising, then, that we think a lot about food, and the thought, of course, is parent to the deed. The more we think about it, the more we are likely to consume.

Hence, one of the big challenges while we diet is to keep our minds off our stomachs. It's not enough to simply tell ourselves to stop thinking about food; we must provide reasonable substitutes.

Keeping busy helps—and it's especially useful when we can occupy our minds as well as our bodies. The diet will go particularly well if you plan it for a time when you will be actively involved in work and projects and non-food-oriented play. It will go particularly poorly if you sit around idly thinking about all the tasty morsels you would enjoy putting into your mouth. Don't allow yourself to be *just* a victim of circumstances—as if you alone were molded by happenstance and your surroundings—but instead try molding circumstances to your benefit.

The I-Like-My-Beer Diet, happily, provides you with assistance. Along with each day's diet, I have included a set of questions and answers to engage your mind, to divert you from hunger pangs and inadvertent exposure to food. These diversions are trivia quizzes about beer—and about all aspects of life as it relates to beer: music and art, sports and money, literature, science, politics, history, the day-to-day aspects of living, and more. If you simply read them straight through, questions and answers both, they'll keep you busy for an hour or three.

Their greatest value will be realized, however, if you take time with them, allotting each set to each day of your diet, pondering each question and each answer, using them as a means for occupying and stimulating your mind. Many of the questions are quite difficult, not meant to be answered so much as to provoke, entertain, and enlighten.

One of the satisfactions in this diet, I hope, is that you will be successful in your attempt to lose weight. An equal satisfaction can be that you also become a more informed, more learned, more enlightened person than you were before. Certainly, that has been my experience as I have accumulated all the Diversions for your inspection.

I would make the following suggestions: Read one question at a time. Ponder its implications and significance (if any) to you personally and to the world in which we live. Let your mind wander freely, not only in terms of the specific answer called for, but also as you may think of related subjects that stimulate your imagination for a while. Discuss the matter with one or more friends. If you find a disagreement, argue it at length. Many of the items are great stimuli for saloon banter, or for sharing knowledge with teenage kids, or a friend or spouse.

When you have completely exhausted all the potential inherent in a question, then—and only then—go on to the answer. Use the same technique with each answer that you do with each question. Remember: the intent is to amuse, entertain, and educate yourself; but—even more important—you want to distract and divert yourself away from food. Be sure to extract full value out of each item.

Save some items for when you will need them most, when you are most likely to be tempted by the refrigerator, or the kitchen cupboard. The Lord's Prayer does not say, "Help us to resist temptation." It was inspired by a greater wisdom than that. Once the temptation is in front you, the battle is 60 percent lost. Instead, the Lord's Prayer says "Lead us not into temptation," Use the Diversions to keep you occupied, to wipe out any awareness of hunger before it can get you into trouble.

ENJOYMENT

Above all, keep your sense of humor alert! There is no way that a diet can be as much fun as your ordinary eating habits; but if you are watchful, you'll find a lot that is amusing, entertaining, and fulfilling—not only with the Diversions, but also with your own behavior and the reactions of other people to you, as they discover you are losing weight while drinking beer.

Wring all the pleasure out of this irony that you can. Enjoy the audacity of dieting in a way uniquely suited to *you*, one that will escape the approval of stuffy nutritional authorities. Remember that while you are losing weight drinking beer, others are attempting to shed pounds consuming yogurt from low-minded cows and sprouts from dank cellars. Wander over to a health food store and observe all the customers who look as though they arrived years too late.

Rejoice in your beer! Human beings need to consume food that has meaning for them. What meaning is there in a rutabaga or turnip? Indeed, what meaning is there in a meal-in-a-glass diet, some noxious liquid in which are recycled all the chalky leavings from grade school blackboards across the land?

Savor the food that you do have, even though there isn't much of it. I have tried to sprinkle the menus each day with spices and flavors that will appeal to a wide variety of beer drinkers, though my taste inevitably will not be identical to yours. Add herbs and spices to suit your own taste, even if you can't change the amounts or kinds of food themselves.

Rather than menus featuring tiny portions of exquisitely flavored gems, I have emphasized large amounts of full-flavored and filling meal components—for at least one meal each day.

To add to your enjoyment, embark on this diet with one or more friends. Compete and see who loses the most weight. Get all contestants to contribute an entry fee, so the winner will get an appropriate prize.

Experiment with new beers, previously unfamiliar to you. Sip with patient joy. Leave guzzling for some other, nondieting time. Take your time. Raise your glass, and toast yourself and the noble dieting adventure upon which you are embarked.

To weight loss, to triumph over adversity, to personal enlightenment . . . and to beer!

A TYPICAL DAY

The pages that follow are designed to help you lose the weight you want. If you are a 180-pounder, an active man or woman regularly on the go, but not specifically doing heavy physical work, you should lose close to 10 pounds without difficulty. If you weigh 135 pounds and do anything more than sit on your rear all day, you should lose 5 pounds or close to it. If you weigh more to start off with, or are more active, you can expect to lose more. If you weigh less and are essentially inactive, you will lose less. That, of course, is if you follow the diet exactly.

The allocation of food throughout the day is as follows:

Breakfast: 100 calories
Small meal: 200 calories
Main meal: 400 calories
Beer: 300 calories

You can move some of the calories around, depending on the peculiarities of your own dietary habits and working conditions, but for best results I would encourage you to stick as closely as possible to my outline.

I assume that most people will have their small meal at lunch and their main meal at supper, but these can be switched, if you wish. If for some reason you can't stand one of the menus suggested (e.g., you are allergic to seafood), you can repeat a meal from another diet day. For instance, feel free to substitute any one main meal for another, or any one small meal for another.

The I-Like-My-Beer Diet allows you to save 300 calories out of 1,000 each day for beer. There is some variation from one brand to another (see Appendix), but we will proceed on the assumption that you will be able to consume two 12-ounce containers of regular beer each day.

When you have those beers is solely a matter of personal preference. I like to have one when I come home from work and then one in the evening, though I will occasionally forfeit one of them so I can have a beer with my main meal. I never have beer with my midday meal on a working day, because I want to keep my thinking as sharp as I can and I also don't want alcohol on my breath when I am seeing patients. Your situation may be different, and you can make adjustments accordingly.

A word about so-called light or low-calorie beers: Light beers generally have at least one-third fewer calories than the brewer's regular label. Therefore, for any given brand, the calorie content of three light beers equals or may even be less than the calorie content of two regular beers. If you wish, you may have *three light beers instead of two regular beers* each day.

Frankly, I prefer the two regular beers, though in some special situations (e.g., a Saturday when I am watching the game on the tube or when I am eating such highly spiced food that the taste of the beer is not quite so important), I will switch to the low-cal stuff.

Remember, however, *always have one 12-ounce glass of water before each beer*, whether it is regular or light.

Recognizing that successful dieting is very much influenced by social circumstances and the organization of your working day, I have given you three alternatives for every small and main meal. The first alternative (the Chef's Choice) assumes that either you or someone in your family likes or is willing to cook and has some basic cooking skills. This option will allow you to mold your daily intake exactly to the demands of the diet, and will give you the widest range of flavors and tastes over the twelve days.

Each recipe is designed for one person only. If you are cooking for more than one, simply multiply the ingredients by the number of people being served. As you start this diet, it is extremely useful to have one or more nonstick pans, particularly an eight-inch frying pan. A mere tablespoon of cooking oil, at 120 calories, is the caloric equivalent of 10 ounces of most beers, so anything you can do to limit the amount of oil or fat you use in cooking will result in sudsy dividends.

The second alternative (the Restaurant Plate) is based on the fact that many of us are required, either by business or social circumstances, to take some meals each week at a restaurant.

Yes, you can follow the I-Like-My-Beer Diet at restaurants, but it will require an extra measure of care in selecting the restaurant and an extra measure of discipline at the table. *Stay away from fast food places*, unless they have a salad bar. Otherwise, they are Fat City! Remember that all restaurant meals in this diet are interchangeable in caloric value—small meal for small meal, and main meal for main meal—so if you don't have, for example, a Japanese restaurant in your area, feel free to substitute from another day.

Once in the restaurant, the first thing to do is ask for a *big* glass (beer glass size, or 12 full ounces) of water, and drink it before doing anything else. Ask the waiter to remove the bread and butter from the table. If you can't do that because of others who are dining with you, prepare to be virtuous. Remember to follow the instructions for each day's diet, and do not have dessert.

While each day's diet allows you to eat in a restaurant, your best shot for losing weight over the twelve days will be to keep your number of restaurant visits to a minimum. While the restaurant menu items I suggest are likely to fall within our calorie limits, it is also possible that they will not. No one knows what the chef will put into your meal, sometimes not even the chef. Unmeasured or reckless use of butter, cooking oils, and starches can botch your diet without your even knowing it. Read the words of caution included in my comment about each restaurant meal.

The third alternative recognizes that many of us either don't like to cook or because of other factors are unable to do so, and additionally are prevented by circumstances from dining out. This option (the Brown Bag) assumes only that you have available a microwave oven or some other heating device and a few utensils. While the Brown Bag may seem like a much compromised eating situation, it is actually an ideal way to approach the diet. You will be exposed only to the food you have with you and therefore temptation will be at a minimum. You will have the perfect opportunity to focus on each day's trivia questions and answers as well, brown-bagging either with a friend or alone.

The brown bag approach is therefore highly recommended, whether you do it at home or at work. The brand-name items have been carefully selected and are therefore much safer in terms of calories than an unpredictable restaurant—and marginally safer than cooking yourself, especially if you are the sort of person for whom time spent at the refrigerator and stove is a time of great temptation. All the brown bag menus are for the entire portion of the item listed, on the assumption that willpower is not your strong suit, and restricting yourself to only part of a portion already in front of you is unlikely and perhaps impossible. Brand-name items, however, are changing all the time, reflecting the availability of ingredients and recipe changes, and some items are not sold in all areas consistently. If you have to substitute, stick to our calorie guidelines for each meal.

A word about parties. Unless your willpower is substantially better than mine, parties will be as destructive to your dieting efforts as they have been to mine. While I am dieting, I try to avoid them. Small dinners or gatherings with friends are manageable, however, when they understand that I'm on a diet and won't try to subvert my efforts. People vary enormously in the amount of sympathy and helpfulness you can expect from them in this matter. However, many hosts and hostesses can become very enthusiastic about something as zany as the I-Like-My-Beer Diet, and going over the trivia quizzes with a willing group of friends in a party atmosphere can be a lot of fun. Call your host or hostess in advance to make certain that they will be on your side.

Most of us find weekends the hardest times for dieting, so for best results I would suggest you organize the twelve days of your diet to start on a Monday and end on a Friday. With only one weekend in the middle of the ordeal, that will give you the best shot at losing the most weight. However, if you ordinarily work Saturdays and Sundays, as I often do, you may wish to juggle the starting day.

Finally, let me suggest you save your empty beer bottles or cans as you go along. Stack them prominently on some easily visible shelf. It will be gratifying for you to see a full case of empties accumulate as your diet reaches its successful conclusion.

Good luck! I hope this diet works as well for you as it has for me. Come to think of it, I've put on weight lately. I'll go on the diet again with you!

DIET
·&·
DIVERSIONS

DAY 1 DIET

Most readers will be starting this diet on a Monday. Mondays, of course, stink. It's back to the working grind again after a weekend of pleasurable abandon, including, most likely, some overdoing it with food and beverages. Start your day by stepping on the scale. There's a cheery idea. Remember, the higher the reading now, the more pounds you are likely to lose in the days ahead.

Mondays are great times for going on diets. Did you know that more than a quarter of the people who drop dead from strokes or heart attacks succumb on Mondays? It's true. In some studies, up to 43 percent of the sudden deaths had their ticket punched on this very day. Survive Monday, and the odds shift significantly in your favor!

After getting off the scale, be sure to take your multivitamin and your thiamine tablet. Swallow them with a good 12 ounces of water.

Here is the program for today:

BREAKFAST:

Breakfast is deliberately a bit skimpy, designed to get you into a foul mood right off the bat. What better time to be a grouch than Monday morning? Remember, your reward for this deprivation will come later in the day.

The Menu   Vegetable Juice or Tomato Juice
(12 ounces)
Coffee or Tea (as much as you like)

MIDMORNING:

For your coffee break, drink as much coffee or tea (no sugar, milk, or cream) as you wish. Skip any doughnuts or sweet rolls. There's no need to be nice about it.

LUNCH:

Your small meal for today is in keeping with Monday's spartan program, but a distinct improvement in tastiness over breakfast. If you can't stand one of the ingredients on the menu, feel free to exchange today's lunch for one on any other day. Their caloric values are all roughly equal.

Be sure to have a 12-ounce glass of water before your meal.

If you are eating in a situation where you might easily be tempted to have more than the prescribed dietary allowance, bring out the Diversion Quiz for today—or save it for later in the day, if you wish.

The Menu   Chef's Choice Lunch: Asparagus
Zingers

This is a great dish, whether you are eating at home or if you cook at home and keep lunch refrigerated for you at work. It's a one-dish meal, filling and quite tasty. Enjoy!

18–20 asparagus spears, cooked till wilted, then
   chopped
 3 tablespoons canned jalapeno peppers,
   drained (or more if you wish)
 3 scallions
 ½ large tomato
 2 teaspoons vegetable oil
2–3 teaspoons lemon or lime juice
1–3 garlic cloves
1–2 dashes Worcestershire sauce
  Salt and pepper to taste
8–10 lettuce leaves
3–4 teaspoons pimiento garnish

Put all ingredients except the pimiento and lettuce into a blender and blend until smooth. Spoon 2 large tablespoonsful into each lettuce leaf, top with pimiento for color, and fold the lettuce around the filling. Chill and serve. You can eat these with a fork if you have a dislike of sloppy eats, or you can pick up each lettuce fold with your hands.

The Menu Restaurant Lunch: Manhattan Clam Chowder (1 cup) Shrimp Cocktail 1 Beer (optional)

You never quite know what you'll find in a restaurant, but this menu should round out close to 200 calories (beer excluded), assuming you use only a tablespoon or two of cocktail sauce on the shrimp and manage to have *no* bread, rolls, or crackers. If the shrimp is served on lettuce, be sure to demolish that as well: it's filling and has no calories to speak of. Make sure that your chowder is Manhattan style (red); the

New England style (white) has two or three times as many calories.

If you have a beer for lunch, remember that you are allowed only one more for the day—or two more if all of them are light beers. You can, of course, drink coffee or tea as you like.

The Menu   Brown Bag Lunch: Manhattan Clam Chowder (8 ounces) Shrimp Cocktail (4-ounce size)

This is one of those situations where you can dine as well as a brown bagger as you can out in a restaurant for a business lunch, and the brown bagger has the advantage of not being tempted by all the bread, rolls, and menu goodies.

There are many companies that make each of these products. The Manhattan clam chowder is available in 8-ounce cans from Heinz or Campbell (about 75 calories each). Just dump in a bowl and stick in the microwave, or warm in a pan on a hot plate, if that's what's available. The shrimp cocktail may take a little more effort to find, but is available in many supermarkets and delicatessens (e.g., Sau-Sea brand, 4 ounces, at about 115 calories).

MIDAFTERNOON:

Of course, you can have coffee or tea for your afternoon break—or one of the many one-calorie or no-calorie diet beverages available.

SUPPER:

Well, friend, you've made it through most of the first diet day. You deserve a treat. Supper tonight will be more or less in the British style, which makes a beer from the United Kingdom a natural to accompany the meal. Try a Bass or a Watney or whatever else you are moved to sample from your local beer merchant. If you wish, have the beer before dinner, as a token acknowledgment of the cocktail hour. Remember to have a full glass (12 ounces) of water first.

For tonight, imagine that you are Pierce Synnott traveling on a British train in 1936. It's the dining car on the 5:20 from Euston on November 6, and the chef is a magician:

> If the soup was an English lady, the sole was a true English man, fat and tough withal, and browned to a manly tan; in the melted butter swam a few specks of parsley, adding that aphrodisiac quality required to relieve the heavier substance of the fish. With this my Guinness was served—statesman among drinks, that can keep his head and has none of that tiredness which may overcome a milk stout in the course of a long railway journey.

Of course, we aren't going to do any swimming in butter while we're on the diet, but there's nothing wrong with fillet of sole. If you want, you can have Guinness (at 167 calories per 11.4 ounces, it's only a little more fattening than your average beer), but we'll be focusing on the cuisine and brews of Ireland next week, so you may prefer to wait till then.

The Menu   Chef's Choice Dinner: Fillet of Sole, Pub Style

Here's a dish that is a meal in itself, filling and delicious to boot. It's also extremely easy to prepare, so you will have plenty of time left for the Diversion Quiz.

⅔ pound sole fillets
2 scallions, chopped (an equivalent amount of chopped parsley may be substituted)
6 mushrooms, sliced
1 tablespoon bread crumbs
2 zucchini, peeled and sliced
  Salt and pepper to taste
¼ cup dry white wine
2 tablespoons lemon juice
2 tablespoons chopped watercress

Place the fillets in a coverable oven dish, or on a large piece of heavy-duty aluminum foil, if you wish (be sure to raise the edges so the liquid will be retained). Pour wine over the fish and tuck the zucchini around the edges. Sprinkle the other ingredients on top. Then cover the dish, or fold and seal the foil; bake in a preheated oven at 350° for 20 minutes.

The Menu   Restaurant Dinner: Broiled or Grilled Fish Green Vegetables

A fish restaurant is usually a good place to eat when you are being careful about your caloric intake. Stick to fish that is broiled, poached, or grilled, hopefully with a minimum of butter. Avoid cream sauces and any bread products. The more careful you are about this sort of nonsense, the more successful your diet will be. Fish that are lowest in calories include sole, haddock, flounder, and cod. Salmon is, of course, one of God's special gifts to His humble servants on earth, but unfortunately so rich that it must be excluded from our diet.

The term *green vegetables* here refers to any low-calorie veggies. If they are green they are probably safe (excluding avocados), but the permissible group also includes cauliflower, carrots, radishes, tomatoes, summer squash, and mushrooms. Stay away from butter and sauces, of course. Instead, season with lemon juice (there should be plenty available at any fish restaurant) or Worcestershire sauce.

The Menu   Brown Bag Dinner: Fish Dinner

Fortunately, there are lots of frozen fish dinners available, and most of them are fairly low-cal. Avoid those that are batter-dipped and french-fried, however, because they give you twice as many calories as you should have. Both Morton and Banquet put out frozen fish dinners (about 9-oz. size) that give decent food value and fall below our 400-calorie limit. You can jazz the dinner up a bit with lemon juice or some horseradish sauce.

EVENING:

If you have only had one beer so far (or two lights), another of the same awaits your pleasure. Be sure to have a 12-ounce glass of water first. Relax, settle in with the Diversion Quiz, and enjoy the quiet pleasure of a successful first diet day.

DAY 1 DIVERSIONS

Q. Ale plays a role in a number of Shakespeare's plays—and no wonder, since brewed beverages were the standard fluid consumed with or without meals during his day. Yet it is also true that ale was particularly important to the Shakespeare family in that young Will's father was an ale-conner. What, for heaven's sake, is an ale-conner?

A. Since ale was so important to English well-being, the king was very concerned that its quality and availability be suitable for his subjects. The ale-conner was an official whose job it was to determine the price for ale, as well as to decide whether a specific ale was of sufficient quality to be sold at all. One test used by these worthies was to pour samples of the brew on a bench. The conner, who wore leather breeches, then sat in the puddle for a specific period of time. If there was sugar in the ale, the conner's breeches would stick to the bench, possibly evidence also that the beer was tainted by additives. It depends on what source you read, however. One writer says that if the breeches stick to the bench, that was evidence that the beer was honest. Take your pick.

Q. In 1920, a prominent American brewer who just happened to own the New York Yankees bought Babe Ruth from the Boston Red Sox for $525,000, part of which apparently was a loan to help out the beleaguered Red Sox owner Harry Frazee. Ruth gratified the owner of his new club by popping

54 home runs in his first year, and Yankee attendance more than doubled. Who was the man who owned the Yankees?

A. Jacob Ruppert was a brewer like his father before him, but with a Midas touch. He was one of the relatively small number of brewers rich enough to survive the rigors of Prohibition without much difficulty. However, the company finally folded in 1965. The New York City plant was closed and the brand name was sold to Rheingold. In 1940, however, the Ruppert brewery was one of the six largest in the United States.

Q. What common expression, having to do with attention to detail, is directly derived from English beer-drinking (and -serving) tradition?

A. "Mind your P's and Q's." The expression derives from the pre–cash register days, in which purchases by tavern patrons would be recorded on a board or wall, depending upon whether the customer ordered pints ("P's") or quarts ("Q's"). The tavern keeper would remind the barmaids and customers to "watch your P's and Q's"—that is, don't forget how much money is owed.

Q. In 1978, David Ogilvy published an autobiography that told of his successes in life and, of necessity, his own brilliance, energy, and glamour, which attracted fortune's gifts. Ogilvy was one of the founders of the advertising agency Ogilvy and Mather, and he takes credit for the famous advertisements touting Hathaway shirts (the model with the black eye-patch), Schweppes (Commander Whitehead), Rolls-Royce, and Dove soap, among many. As Ogilvy said: "I doubt whether any copywriter has ever produced so many winners in such a short period." If you know the title of his autobiography, you'll know what nourished this healthy ego in his fledgling years.

A. Ogilvy's father was a dedicated scholar and a rugged partisan of unusual appetites: he ate Coleman's hot mustard by the spoonful. To make his six-year-old son as strong and brainy as himself, he put him on a diet of raw blood (a glassful) daily with calves' brains three times a week, washed down with a bottle of beer. His son's autobiography is entitled *Blood, Brains, and Beer.*

Q. "A nimble waiter brings a large bottle of Murree Export Lager. The hotel is empty; the other guests have risked a punishing journey to Swat in hopes of being received by His Highness, the Wali. You sleep soundly under a tent of mosquito net and are awakened by the fluting of birds for an English breakfast that begins with porridge and ends with a kidney." This passage was taken from a best-selling travel adventure of the mid-1970s by Paul Theroux. What is the name of the book and where does one find Murree Export Lager?

A. Paul Theroux drank his Murree in Peshawar, Pakistan, after disembarking from the Khyber Pass Local, on a trip that had begun long before in London, as recounted in *The Great Railway Bazaar.* After the beer, he rode along broad, sleepy roads under cool trees to the museum, where he had the pleasure of learning how Buddha was conceived: "There is a Graeco-Buddhist frieze in the Peshawar Museum showing Buddha's mother lying on her side and being impregnated through her ribs by what looks like the nozzle of a hot-air balloon suspended over her. In another panel the infant Buddha is leaping from a slit in her side—a birth with all the energy of a broad jump."

Q. We are all children at heart, and so most of us have seen the movie *E.T.*, that heartwarming and whimsical space-age version of *Peter Pan.* One of the most amusing scenes is when the extraterrestrial himself gets drunk on an earthly brew. Many viewers were surprised to see the beer's label so clearly visible on the screen. See if you can remember. What brand of beer got E.T. looped?

A *E.T.* was the movie of the year in 1982, earning $187 million in rental revenues, about triple the figure earned by the number-two film, *Rocky III*. By the end of 1982, *E.T.* had already outsold *Jaws, Raiders of the Lost Ark, The Sound of Music*, and *Gone with the Wind*—and was rapidly creeping up on the all-time leader, *Star Wars*. All these ticket holders watched E.T. swig Coors, the cult favorite of many Western beer drinkers. Coors itself is no slouch as a money-maker; it is the seventh-largest beer producer in the world and fifth-largest in the United States.

Q. We make such a fuss about alcohol today that it is sometimes difficult to keep matters in perspective. In May 1904, the editor of a famous women's magazine made the following observation: "A mother who would hold up her hands in holy horror at the thought of her child drinking a glass of beer, which contains from two to five percent alcohol, gives to that child with her own hands a potent medicine that contains from 17 to 44 percent alcohol." What women's magazine still being published and still with a hefty circulation was thereby put on record, endorsing beer for children over patent medicines?

A. The quotation is directly from a Budweiser advertisement of the time, but first appeared in a full-page article in the Ladies' Home Journal under the by-line of its editor, Edward Bok. He went on to say: "In connection with this list, think of beer, which contains only from two to five percent alcohol, while some of these 'bitters' contain 10 times as much, making them stronger than whiskey, far stronger than Sherry or Port, with Claret or Champagne way behind." To put the matter in a more modern perspective, here are the alcohol contents of commonly used over-the-counter cough and cold syrups: Novahistine, 10 percent; Formula 44, 10 percent; Nyquil, 25 percent.

Q. Nowadays, most folks are familiar with George Killian's Irish Red, a specialty beer produced by Coors, which suffers, in my judgment, from being an 11-ounce commodity in a 12-ounce industry. However, there was another Kilian (one *l*), a St. Kilian, who was important to the brewing industry. Who was this man and what did he do?

A. St. Kilian died a martyr's death in A.D. 689, perhaps a natural consequence of an Irishman's presuming to do missionary work in the Wurzburg area of Germany. Nonetheless, St. Kilian's work bore fruit, and in the following century, tiny Wurzburg was elevated by St. Boniface to a bishopric. Thousands of pilgrims came to visit the shrine of St. Kilian. It was, in part, to serve all these pilgrims that the brewery in Wurzburg was developed. Wurzburger Hofbrau has been a popular import in the United States since the 1800s, when its fame was enhanced by special attention lavished on it by Luchow's restaurant in New York City.

Q. In Nicholas Blake's whodunit *There's Trouble Brewing*, the brewing industry has a hard time of it. One brewer gets polished off in the wort and another brewer appears to be the culprit. Fortunately, the gentleman detective, Nigel Strangeways, is on the case and helps to solve the mystery. But what, for heaven's sake, is the wort?

A. The principal ingredients in beer are water, malt, and hops, which are all boiled together in huge vats to make a vast soup. This bubbling, frothy, smelly, rich concoction is called the wort. When all the ingredients are blended together, the wort is cooled, the yeast is added, and fermentation begins. You can imagine what happens to a corpse that sojourns for an hour or more in the boil. Not much left except the bones. Of course, all the wags in the pub thought it added more body to the beer.

Q. All right, art fans, here's one for *you*. Impressionist Édouard Manet, the scandal of Paris for many years because of some of his alarmingly realistic nudes (Napoleon III called one of his paintings "an offense against modesty"), also created many works in which beer was a prominent subject. One of Manet's few works to achieve popularity in his own lifetime is *Le Bon Bock*, which features a portly Dutch-style beer drinker. His last major work, *Bar at the Folies Bergère* (1882), lets us clearly see the label on two bottles of beer, of a brand that is still consumed today and known by savvy beer drinkers the world over. What is that beer?

A. On either side of the barmaid, one can see labels sporting the red triangle characteristic of Bass & Co. Pale Ale, a major British export then, and now the product of one of the world's largest brewing companies. The red triangle, by the by, was the first registered trademark in Britain, issued under the Trade Marks Act of 1890.

Q. Interested in botany? The old Roman name for the common hop was *Lupus sarictarius*, meaning "like a wolf among the sheep," apparently referring to the fact that the hop grew wild among the willows. The current Latin name for the common hop is *Humulus lupulus*, indicating both genus and species. To what botanical family does the hop belong?

A. The hop belongs to the family *Cannabinaceae* and, as with the marijuana plant, it is the resin-producing female plant that has great commercial value. Only the catkins of the seedless female hops are used for beer. The seedy male hops are too bitter. Seedless marijuana is known as sensimilla, derived from the Spanish meaning *without seed*.

Q. From the thirteenth century for several hundred years afterward, the work of brewing in England was largely the province of women, the alewives—perhaps because it was largely a domestic or kitchen-based operation. The alewives had reputations for being a very colorful and carefree lot—which meant, of course, that the king's officials tried to keep a close watch on them. What was the punishment for an alewife who fraudulently mislabeled the quality or quantity of the brew she sold?

A. Alewives who were first-time or minor offenders were customarily fined, but after repeated fines they might be pilloried, so that the beer-drinking mob could have at the troublemakers, throwing rotten cabbages and tomatoes and other sundries. In some parts, the ducking stool was also used. A paragraph from the *London Evening Post* (1745) described one incident: "Last week a woman that keeps the Queens Head Alehouse at Kingston Surrey was ordered by the Court to be ducked . . . and was accordingly placed in the chair and ducked in the river Thames under Kingston Bridge, in the presence of 2,000 or 3,000 people."

Q. The beer barrel has been a source of inspiration for many. Where would the "Beer Barrel Polka" be without it? As with barrels of all kinds, it occasionally serves as furniture or as a planter, and it has been used as a hurdle to be overcome by ice skaters doing stunts. What is the most famous and dangerous barrel stunt of all time?

A. For a number of years, in the middle of the century, a popular challenge for daredevils was to ride over Niagara Falls in a barrel. A number of people killed themselves in this fashion. In September 1948, William (Red) Hill, Jr., succeeded in shooting the Lower Rapids in the Niagara River. On emerging from the barrel, his first words were: "Somebody give me a beer."

Q. So many treasures of uniqueness and excellence have been lost to the blandness of contemporary taste, the economics of scale inherent in corporate brewing, the dictates of politics, and trade and tariff wars. However, improbably, Russian Imperial Stout is still being brewed commercially by the Courage & Barclay Company in London. What is Russian Imperial Stout?

A. As long ago as 1795, Catherine the Great ordered vast amounts of what came to be called Russian Imperial Stout for her own consumption and that of her court. This remarkable brew, composed only of water, malt, and hops, is twice as strong as Guinness, so strong in fact that the one-third-pint "nip" bottles are said to be the alcoholic equivalent of four whiskeys. It is aged for two months in casks and for another year in bottles before leaving the brewer's cellars. With careful storage and handling, the beer will continue to age 7–10 years or more. Grants Brewery in Yakima, Washington, reportedly makes a fine Russian Imperial Stout, though I have yet to taste it.

Q. You know beer, so you know the difference between lager, ale, and pilsener. What, exactly, *is* the difference?

A. Lager is the type of beer most of us drink, accounting for the overwhelming majority of American and German beer consumed. It tends to be light and dry in taste, brewed with a bottom-fermenting yeast. Pilsener is a variety of lager, referring to a style originating in Pilsen, Bohemia, usually implying the use of Czechoslovakian hops. Ale is brewed with a different yeast entirely, a top-fermenting variety, at slightly higher temperatures, in the British style. Usually the taste is more tart and it is not quite so crisp and sparklingly clear in a glass as lager.

DAY 2 DIET

Welcome to Tuesday, the second-worst day of the week. Tuesday is the kind of day that the stock market would pick for its biggest plunge—as it did on October 29, 1929—or that a scoundrel like Bruno Hauptmann would choose to kidnap Charles A. Lindbergh, Jr. (March 1, 1932). Tuesday is so bad that even the U.S. government picked it for its recommended meatless day during World War II, to help compensate for wartime shortages.

Cheer up. None of those things are likely to happen to you. You got through yesterday, and with the help of the malt, you'll survive today. Start the day with 12 ounces of water, a multivitamin, and your thiamine tablet.

BREAKFAST:

Contrary to what the bacon-and-egg folks would have you believe, breakfast is *not* necessarily the most important meal of the day. Importance—when it comes to timing your various repasts—is largely a matter of personal values and habits. For the average person on the average weekday, breakfast is the meal with the least personal value, largely because it is usually eaten rapidly—without much opportunity for savoring flavors or textures—and while you are as yet barely awake. It is therefore a meal in which one can cut down on calories without an intolerable psychic impact. Our menu today is spartan without being sadistic.

The Menu **Puffed Rice (1 cup), seasoned with cinnamon and artificial sweetener**
Skim milk (¼ cup)
Vegetable Juice (6 ounces)
Coffee or Tea (ad lib)

MIDMORNING:

Drink as much coffee or tea as your bladder and caffeine-sensitivity will allow. Again, skip all munchies.

LUNCH:

This is the middle of the second day. You are doing extremely well, despite the odds. With your morale on an even keel, we'll do a soup number for lunch; filling, yet not too chewy. Drink 12 ounces of water first.

The Menu **Chef's Choice Lunch:** **Egg Drop Soup**
Tomato-Cucumber Vinaigrette

Both of these dishes are best served fresh, if you have a kitchen handy. However, the soup can be prepared in advance and carried to work in a thermos—or rewarmed in a microwave. The salad, of course, is easily transported in a refrigerator dish.

EGG DROP SOUP·

1 cup chicken broth
2 scallions, thinly sliced
4 mushrooms, thinly sliced
2 small slices fresh ginger
1 egg, beaten
Salt and pepper to taste

The chicken broth is best made from cubed concentrate or a packet of bouillon. If you use canned broth, be sure to skim off the fat before you dump the liquid in the pan. Fresh ginger is a zesty seasoning to keep around and very low-cal; simply store it in the freezer and slice off chunks as needed. To make the soup, heat the liquid; then add scallions, mushrooms, and ginger. Remove from the heat when the liquid reaches a boil, and slowly stir in the egg. Serve promptly, with salt and pepper to taste.

TOMATO-CUCUMBER VINAIGRETTE

2 medium tomatoes, sliced
½ medium cucumber, peeled and sliced
2 tablespoons low-cal Italian salad dressing

Sprinkle veggies with the dressing; chill and serve.

The Menu   Restaurant Lunch: Chicken or Shrimp Wonton Soup *or* Egg Drop Soup

Chinese restaurants are now available in most cities and towns and are good places to stop for light lunches, if you can be selective in your choices. Order a bowl of any of the above, but don't take any refills. Caloric values can vary widely from one restaurant to another, but these soups should fall below our limit. The broth or the soup should be thin enough so you can see individual constituents floating in it. Drink as much tea as you like, and treat yourself to a single fortune cookie. If you are having a beer, consider an exotic Asian brand, like Tsingtao from China, Amarit from Thailand, or Tiger from Singapore.

The Menu   Brown Bag Lunch: Hot Soup
Coffee, Tea, or
Diet Beverage

If you want to stay in tune with the Asian motif of the business lunch, Campbell makes a reasonable wonton soup that weighs in at about 100 calories per 10 ¾-ounce can. Be careful of the various Oriental noodle meal-in-a-cup soup mixes; most of them don't list caloric values, and those that do may run over 300 calories. Actually, practically any noncream soup made by Campbell is a good bet. Check the cans; all of them list calorie content. Remember, our luncheon limit is 200 calories.

MIDAFTERNOON:

Have a diet beverage, carbonated water, tea, or coffee. If your stomach starts to complain, turn to the Diversions for a quiz break.

SUPPER:

If you toughed it out over lunch, you can look forward to a glass of beer during the cocktail hour. First do the glass-of-water number, and then choose some fine lager beer to delight you. We're having German food for dinner, in large quantities, so a small celebration is in order. As H. L. Mencken observed, "Sauerkraut is good for your innards, cleans up all the germs, and leaves you as fresh as when your father first left a souvenir with your mother."

**The Menu   Chef's Choice Dinner: Frankfurters
with
mustard
Sauerkraut**

Making sauerkraut the old-fashioned way requires a good two weeks or more, a big barrel or keg, lots of cabbage and salt, and a scattering of apples or grapes for flavoring. Like beer, sauerkraut is a fermented food—and fermentation is not to be rushed. Under the circumstances, it makes sense to let the food purveyors do most of our work for us.

Take any brand of canned sauerkraut and place a cup or two in a pan. Kraut runs 30–60 calories a cup, and you can therefore eat your fill. Add two tablespoons of crushed caraway seeds. Slice up two frankfurters (use chicken or turkey franks and save a few extra calories—or use the standard variety, if you prefer) and add them to the pan. Heat just to boiling, remove, and serve with the mustard of your choice. An alternate method is to grill the frankfurters separately, thereby keeping the tastes more distinct, but losing some juices in the process.

The Menu   Restaurant Supper: Sauerkraut plus careful selection

If work or a social gathering takes you to a German restaurant, you need to proceed carefully indeed if you are to avoid losing ground—meaning gaining weight. Avoid all the things you would ordinarily love to salivate over, and save them for the next visit after the diet. The best bet is to fill up on sauerkraut. If the restaurant has ordinary frankfurters in the standard size, you can safely have two—but make sure that nothing else is added to your plate except green vegetables. If frankfurters are lacking, ask for a single lean sausage or, failing that, a salad and a bowl of soup—with, of course, the sauerkraut on the side.

The Menu   Brown Bag Special: Sauerkraut and Frankfurters

Luck is with you today. You can eat just as well as the folks on their expense accounts. Empty a can or jar of sauerkraut into a bowl, place two frankfurters on top, heat in a microwave, and serve with your favorite mustard.

EVENING:

If so far today you have had only one regular beer or two light beers, you can have another of the same while relaxing this evening. Remember to have 12 ounces of water before the beer. Finish up the Diversion Quiz—and so to bed

DAY 2 DIVERSIONS

Q. An extraordinary tribute it is, to be sure, to have one's portrait and name adorn the label of a world-famous beer. Einbeck Beer has been brewed since 1351, and Einbeck was once the most famous brewing city in the world. Shortly after bottling beer for export to the United States, Einbeck honored the world-famous leader of a Protestant denomination by putting out a beer in his honor. Who was that person?

A. Einbeck has been called the Beer of Martin Luther, not only because his picture has graced one of its labels, but also because he was given some as a wedding present by the city of Wittenberg—and a full barrel as a gift from the Duke of Brunswick, to fortify him during the Diet of Worms. No, the Diet of Worms was not an early fad diet. A diet in those days was a meeting or, by extension, the body that convened the meeting. The Diet of Worms in 1521 was held in the hope of reconciling Luther's teachings with those of Roman Catholicism. In that regard, it failed. Luther was condemned as a heretic—and so transpired an important milestone in the development of Protestantism.

Q. In 1913–14, a prominent American beer drinker and wordsmith was invited to write advertising material for the brewers' association. He claimed, "I was offered $30,000 cash, deposited in bank to my order, to write anti-Prohibition speeches for the illiterates in the two Houses of Congress.

The money is enough to make me dizzy, but I fear it would mean contact with brewers and such-like swine." Who is it who loved beer so much and brewers so little?

A. H. L. Mencken's favorite beverage was beer, but he maintained that there was no alcoholic beverage that he would turn away (he was, he said, "omni-bibulous"). One day he drank only ten beers and was thoroughly ashamed of himself because he felt full and unable to consume more. He believed that most of the problems attributed to overeating were actually a result of underdrinking. He reportedly held William Howard Taft (the twenty-seventh president and tenth chief justice of the United States) in awe because he was one of the few people who could outeat and outdrink him.

Q. Many folks who admire fine craftwork like German beer steins. They come in an enormous range of shapes, sizes, colors, and designs. The word *stein* itself means *stone*, and is derived from the fact that the first steins, created some 500 years ago, were made of stoneware or earthenware. Why do steins have those damn lids that keep getting in a beer drinker's way?

A. Anything so dumb as the lid on the beer stein *has* to be related to some outmoded governmental regulation and so, of course, it is. In the late sixteenth century, Germany was plagued with swarms of insects that were forever attracted to the aromatic and tasty beer. Officials decreed that all drinking vessels should have lids, so now 400 years later you can still bump your nose into one.

Q. Up until the mid-ninteenth century, American beers were basically beverages in the British tradition: ales, strong beers and porters. After that time, lager made its appearance and gradually became dominant. Why then?

A.   Well, there was an enormous influx of Germans, for whom lager beer was as natural as air itself. Germans had been emigrating to America in dribs and drabs throughout the eighteenth century, but the trickle turned to a deluge with the German economic and political instability of the nineteenth century, especially with the uprisings of 1848. A more technical, companion explanation is that lager beer was brewed with a yeast that fermented at the bottom of the vat, instead of the top, as with ale yeasts. Yeast, of course, is a living product, a biological enzyme, and this particular one was so fragile that it could survive, even with refrigeration, for a maximum of four weeks. It was only with the development of fast clipper ships, capable of making the voyage in three weeks, that lager yeast could be transported to the New World.

Q.   If your school days were like mine, you encountered at least one beer-chugging contest. It's not the brightest part of an education, but a necesary rite of passage for lots of us idiots. What is the fastest that any human being can chug a gallon of beer?

A.   Up until 1972, according to *The Great Canadian Beer Book*, the record was held by an Australian, at 6 minutes 45 seconds. In that year, an incredible new world record was set by David Arsenault of Dalhousie, New Brunswick, in Canada. He quaffed a gallon in 3 minutes 35 seconds, and this *astounding* time included a one-minute penalty for spillage.

Q.   Here is a wonderful classic of political oratory from November 8, 1923: "There is nothing to fear," he cried. "We have the friendliest intentions. For that matter, you've no cause to grumble, you've got your beer!" What famous demagogue made the statement, and where?

A.   The time was almost 9 P.M. on November 8, 1923. This was the Beer Hall Putsch, and Adolf Hitler had just surprised the crowd with the announcement "The National Revolution has begun!" When Hitler took the three leaders of the assembled crowd into another room for private discussions, Hermann Göring was left with 3,000 thirsty burghers who were becoming increasingly resentful of having been commandeered at gunpoint. Göring therefore went to the rostrum in order to quiet the sullen crowd, and made his classic statement. The Putsch was premature, Göring was wounded, and Hitler was imprisoned—for a while. Later Göring fathered the Gestapo and became president of the Reichstag and head of the Luftwaffe.

Q.   These days we're very concerned about the purity of what we eat and drink. Aside from those related to religious practices, one of the oldest laws still in effect governing the purity of food and drink concerns beer and brewing. Which one is that?

A.   In 1516, Wilhelm IV, Duke of Bavaria, decreed the Reinheitsgebot (the Bavarian Pledge of Purity), specifying that the only acceptable components of beer are water, malt, and hops. This standard is still maintained in all of West Germany, Luxembourg, and Switzerland for their domestic brews, though only Bavaria still observes the same standard for its export beers as well. Some of the smaller new breweries in the U.S. adhere to the standards set forth in the Reinheitsgebot, but of course they are not required by law to do so. Christian Moerlein beer, brewed by Hudepohl in Cincinnati, recently received certification by the appropriate West German laboratory, becoming the first U.S. beer to be officially so recognized.

Q.   Alcoholics and drunks give drinking a bad name. However, when the alcoholic is portrayed by Paul Newman, the effect isn't entirely negative—even in the slick, choppy, simplistic movie *The Verdict.* As down-and-nearly-out lawyer Frank Galvin, Newman downs a lot of booze while going on to win a $5 million malpractice verdict (the film doesn't specify the amount, but the book by Barry Reed does)—of which one-third goes to him. While most of what the actor swallows is generic beer and whiskey, at least one beer label is clearly visible in Newman's hand. What is the beer?

A. In addition to having beer with an egg in it for breakfast, Newman is filmed opening and drinking from a can of Budweiser. On special occasions, he orders Bushmill's Irish whiskey, but his regular beverage seems to have been draft beer. Boston, the film's principal locale, was home to more breweries than Milwaukee up until Prohibition; now it has none. However, Massachusetts has the distinction of allowing a higher specified alcohol content in its beer (12 percent) than any other state allows.

Q. Brewing as a domestic art has long been practiced by women, but commercial brewing has been dominated by men. Nonetheless, in 1975 a woman passed her brewmaster's exam in Germany with the highest score among all competitors. This is a toughie—almost impossible—but highest points if you can guess. Who is that woman?

A. Sister Doris, a twenty-seven-year-old Franciscan nun, aced out all competition in her exam and went on to become brewmaster of the Mallersdorfer Klosterbrauerei, where she is doing God's work for our earthly benefit.

Q. No matter what your favorite brand of imported beer may be, it is unlikely to be of French origin—though Kronenbourg from Alsace is quite popular. The French brewing industry has never achieved the international stature of the French wine industry. Yet the irony remains that the father of modern brewing is a Frenchman. Who is that man?

A. Up until the late nineteenth century, brewing was a very chancy business. Some batches turned out beautifully, and others "went bad." While some brewers had much better luck along these lines than others, there was relatively little understanding of why this was so. Louis Pasteur's contribution was to demonstrate that "bad" or "diseased" batches of fermented beverages were caused by bacteria—and that those bacteria could be inactivated or killed by steaming (or what came to be known as pasteurization), which meant heating the beverages to 150–170 degrees. Pasteur's original work was proposed as a means of preserving wine and beer, and for that he is known as "the Father of Modern Brewing." The usefulness of pasteurization for milk was discovered later.

Q. West Germans drink more beer per capita than any other national group, and a fussy lot they are, too. They have a right to be chauvinistic about their country's diversity and quality of beer (and they are, of course), so one would expect them to be highly selective when drinking beers of the other countries. What is far and away the number-one imported beer in Germany?

A. The original pilsener beer from Czechoslovakia, Prazdroj Urquel, easily outsells all others. Germany brews many pilsener-style beers, but somehow none can match the original product. The town of Pilsen is in Bohemia, which currently is located in Czechoslovakia, though of course Germany has annexed it from time to time. Pilsener beers boast a remarkable hoppiness that stimulates the palate—making the beverage a popular aperitif, as well as an accompaniment to meals.

Q. Most beer worthy of the name is brewed from malted barley, though through history practically all grains have been malted for brewing purposes. The most famous beer made in part from wheat is Berliner Weisse, a light and even champagne-like beer sometimes more appreciated by wine lovers than beer lovers. The name means *white* in German, but the unadulterated product is a golden color. Actually, however, when you order it in a Berlin drinking establishment, the Weisse will be layered over or mixed with one of two syrups, which will turn the beer either red or green. What are these syrups?

A. The red syrup (called Schuss) is raspberry extract, and the green (called Waldermeister) is essence of woodruff. Some say that these flavors antedated the use of hops as a flavoring agent. Woodruff has been touted as a tonic, good for the heart and liver, among other things. The red and green colors and their attendant flavors take some getting used to for beer drinkers accustomed to shades of gold and brown.

Q. Paul Theroux's great railway journey through Asia in the early 1970s was mostly hot and dirty work, and a lot of beer was necessary to sustain him on his journey. He searched for it in Sirpur, just over the border of Andhra Pradesh, where the Grand Trunk Express ground to a halt. He managed to find three bottles of warm beer in Villapuram, where the local to Rameswaram changed engines. He rejoiced in a quiet beer with an old friend, after getting off the Golden Arrow in Kuala Lumpur. But it was all worth it, because he managed to learn, among other things, where Cain and Abel are buried. Highest marks if you can guess both the country and the town.

A. This may be difficult to accept, but it is also difficult to disprove. According to local legend, when Adam and Eve were booted out of the Garden of Eden, they went to Sri Lanka. That's why the chain of seven islands across the Palk Strait (which separates India from Ceylon) is called Adam's Bridge. Anyhow, Cain and Abel apparently ended up on the other side of the strait, in Rameswaram, India, which is where they found their final rest. According to Theroux, "The tombs were identical: parallel blocks of crumbling stone on which lizards darted and the green twine of tropical weeds had knotted. I tried to appear reverential, but could not suppress my disappointment at seeing what looked like the foundations of some folly concocted in the Public Works Department."

Q. You probably know that the best-selling beer in the world is Budweiser, brewed by Anheuser-Busch, with corporate offices headquartered in St. Louis, Missouri. What is the origin of the name Budweiser?

A. Budweiser is derived from Budvar beer, a legendary brew from the city of Ceske Budejovice in Bohemia, which is also known by the German name "Budweis." This "Budweiser" beer had so many fans that Adolphus Busch used the name when he launched his Bohemian-style Bud in 1876. However, the original Budweiser was popular as early as 1531, when Czechoslovakian King Ferdinand gave it his royal approval, causing it to be labeled "the Beer of Kings." The American version, of course, is known as "the King of Beers."

Q. Attention comrades, fellow travelers, and other politically savvy beer drinkers: What country would you go to in order to drink a beer called "Economic Warfare"? Guessing is encouraged on this question.

A. Thanks to Idi Amin, no doubt, Uganda has named its best beer Economic Warfare. For this little gem we are indebted to Edward Hoagland, who has written, in the guise of a travel book called *African Calliope*, a lovely little treatise on how much and what kind of beer Africans drink. In addition to all the home brews, the *merissa* of the Sudan and the *pombe* of West Africa, he writes about Zairean Primus and Makasi, Tusker beer from Nairobi, Khartoum beer from the Sudan capital, and Camel beer (which is not identified as to national origin, but two cases of which he and two companions take in lieu of water on a bumpy trip across the desert to Ethiopia).

DAY 3 DIET

Wednesdays are days for major environmental disasters. Just when the middle of the week lulls you into that false sense that there is hope for the world, Mother Nature really socks it to you with something like the Great San Francisco Earthquake (April 18, 1906) or the meltdown at Three Mile Island (March 28, 1979).

In comparison with such cataclysms as these, a third day of dieting is a mere chill in the wind. Not only can you survive it, you will find the tasty repasts nearly enough to keep your stomach quiet and the trivia quiz particularly enlightening and entertaining.

BREAKFAST:

With all the sauerkraut you had last night, you have probably awakened belching and flatulent. Rather than trying to put out the fires, stoke them for all they are worth. Face the day with your innards aglow. Remember to begin with a multivitamin, your thiamine tablet, and 12 ounces of water.

The Menu   **1 egg, poached or fried in a nonstick pan with ½ teaspoon butter topped with salsa jalapeno for flavor**
Coffee or Tea (as much as you wish)

MIDMORNING:

Soak up the coffee or tea, and avoid any tempting sweet or doughy goodies.

LUNCH:

Wednesday lunch has always seemed to me to be a milestone of sorts. It stands (or sits) squarely in the middle of the workday week, with five half-days down and five yet to go. A luncheon of tasty rabbit food therefore is acceptable as a turning point. Life inevitably must begin to improve—if only because the weekend is quickly approaching. Don't forget your 12 ounces of water.

The Menu   Chef's Choice Lunch: Spinach Salad

If Popeye can eat this, so can you. Actually, spinach salad is one of the most appealing of green salads—and this one is a particularly pleasant low-cal version.

½ pound fresh spinach
Juice of ½ lemon
½ cucumber, peeled and sliced
1 egg, hard-boiled and crumbled
6 mushrooms, sliced
4 green onions, sliced in 1″ segments
2 teaspoons salad oil
2 tablespoons white wine vinegar
¼ teaspoons dry mustard
⅛ teaspoon ground cinnamon
Black pepper, ground or cracked, to taste

Remove the stems from the spinach, wash and drain; cut into 1-inch-wide strips. Place in a bowl and chill; then toss leaves with lemon juice; scatter cucumber, egg, mushrooms, and onions on top. In a separate container, combine the oil, vinegar, mustard, and cinnamon, and stir well. Toss the salad with the dressing, and sprinkle pepper on top.

The Menu   Restaurant Lunch: Spinach Salad

Many restaurants carry this item because it appeals to so many patrons. However, you run a risk here if they add a lot of bacon fat, crumbled bacon, croutons, rich dressings, or extra egg. Try to avoid these extras, loaded with heavy-duty calories, and your salad should weigh in at the 200 calories allocated to our average lunch.

The Menu   Brown Bag Lunch: Mushroom-
Tomato Salad

This is a quick and easy meal and quite tasty. I like it served warm, but it is enjoyable chilled as well:

    ½ pound mushrooms
    1 basket cherry tomatoes
    2 tablespoons diet salad dressing

Rinse the mushrooms under running water; remove the stems from the cherry tomatoes; and place the veggies in a plastic container or ordinary dish. Toss with the salad dressing. If you wish, warm this for 60 seconds in the microwave, or serve as is. Do not clean the mushrooms much in advance of serving; they will get soggy.

MIDAFTERNOON:

Have one or more diet drinks, or stick with coffee or tea, if you prefer.

SUPPER:

Yesterday and the day before, the supper menu borrowed from British and German cuisine. Tonight we'll partake of something American, and what could be a better Yankee dinner than a bucket of steamers? Christopher Morley captured the flavor in his *Travels in Philadelphia*:

> When the cold winds begin to harp and whinney at street corners, and wives go seeking among the camphor balls for our last year's overcoats, you will be glad to resume your acquaintance with a bowl of steaming bivalves, swimming in milk, with little clots of yellow butter twirling in the surface of the broth. An oyster stew, a glass of light beer, and a corn-cob pipe will keep your blue eyes blue to any weather, as a young poet of our acquaintance puts it.

Instead of the oysters, we'll go for clams today—and of course we'll forgo the milk and butter, but other than that, our dinner tonight is practically the same as Morley's. To complement the food, have an American beer, perhaps one of the major national brands you haven't tasted in a while, or a product of one of the smaller regional breweries.

The Menu   Chef's Choice Dinner: Steamed
Clams

Cleaning the bivalves requires a little extra work, but it's worth it. This is a lovely dinner to share with friends, a grand occasion for spirited conversation, and for sharing the challenge of today's trivia quiz. Take your time with each clam and with the broth, too. Not a bad diet meal at all. Simply multiply the ingredients by the number of people to be served.

        2 dozen clams
      3–4 garlic cloves
        1 bay leaf
        1 teaspoon butter
          Juice of 1 lemon
          Water
        ½ teaspoon salt

Use only clams with tightly closed shells, and scrub each thoroughly under cold running water to remove sand. In a good-size kettle, place one inch of water and all the ingredients except the clams. When the water is boiling, add the clams and steam for 5–7 minutes (or only until the shells are open). Serve in the kettle or in a large bowl, add hot sauce if you wish, and don't forget to drink the broth.

The Menu   Restaurant Dinner: Steamed Clams

If you have access to a decent seafood restaurant and these little buggers are in season, a bowl of steamers washed down by your favorite beer simply can't be beat. Remember to forgo all the bread and butter the waiter will try to foist on you. The best dessert is conversation.

The Menu   Brown Bag Dinner: Steamed Clams

Incredibly, clams are available canned, steamed in the shells. Brands include Doxsee and Lord Mott's. Simply crank up the microwave and your dinner awaits you. If you have trouble finding cans of clams in the shell, an alternative is to buy canned whole clams (2 cups make a filling meal at only 250 calories); add lemon juice or Worcestershire sauce, and serve piping hot.

EVENING:

If you haven't had your quota of beers for today, relax wih your favorite brew, and finish the Diversion Quiz.

DAY 3 DIVERSIONS

Q. Beer was the universal beverage of the thirteen colonies, the standard drink in the cities and on most farms as well. What accounts for the popularity of beer over such common liquids as milk or even water?

A. Beer was simply safer to consume. Cow's milk was a notorious source of human ills, particularly of tuberculosis. Water in those pre–public health days was even worse as a source of disease. There was no systematic isolation of drinking supplies from contamination by animal or human waste. Very few cities had reliable and tasty sources of water until the mid-nineteenth century. River water—when it was available—tended to be murky, whether laden with disease or not; time had to be allowed for the mud to settle, and the water was likely to remain hazy even then. Rainwater required roof cisterns to collect it, and supplies still tended to be seasonal. Spring water tended to be inaccessible for many, and carrying it much distance was a drag. Beers, on the other hand, were not only yeasty and nutritious, they were overwhelmingly disease-free, due in part to the stabilizing and antibacterial function of alcohol, but also to the boiling phase that is a necessary part of beer's manufacture. Think of the thirteen colonies the next time you are in a country where the *touristas* is a problem, and you'll choose to drink beer instead of tap water.

Q. The top beer-drinking nations, as measured by per capita consumption, are mostly in Europe. In order, they are: West

Germany (1), Belgium (2), Czechoslovakia (3), Luxembourg (6), Denmark (7), Ireland (8), East Germany (9), Great Britain (10), Austria (11), The Netherlands (14), Switzerland (15), Hungary (16), Sweden (17), Finland (18), and Bulgaria (19). The South Pacific is also well represented, with Australia and New Zealand in the fourth- and fifth-highest spots. Which three countries in the Americas are also among the top twenty beer-drinking nations?

A. Canada and the United States are, respectively, in the twelfth and thirteenth places, Venezuela (surprise!) is number twenty. Other leaders in the Americas include Mexico (24), Brazil (27), and Colombia (29). (These figures vary from year to year, but this list is representative.)

Q. Everyone knows that the Puritans were . . . well, puritanical, meaning that they were against pleasure as an end in itself . . . and one might easily assume on this account that they didn't drink beer. One would, however, be wrong. Beer was a crucial provision on the *Mayflower*—so much a necessity, in fact, and so popular, that the dwindling supplies resulted in this intrepid group of settlers giving up hopes of reaching their initial destination, instead accepting for their residence land near their initial landfall of Cape Cod. Where would the Pilgrims have chosen to land had they not run out of beer?

A. They had hoped to settle near "Hudson's River," but because of the uncertainties of navigation and the fickle wind, they hit land north of their initial target. The ship's master and his crew dumped their peculiar passengers at the first opportunity so they could hoard their remaining and much depleted beer supply for the long passage home. The sailors depended on beer to prevent scurvy, when citrus fruits were not available. Whether the beer of that time actually contained enough vitamin C to be of much use is not clear.

Q. In 1970, a very funny book was published about the advertising industry, called *From Those Wonderful Folks Who Gave You Pearl Harbor*, written by a guy named Jerry Della Femina. The man had nothing nice to say about beer or beer drinkers, and almost nothing nice to say about beer advertisements. He suffered from the same glibness of tongue, limited scope, and superficial judgment that unfortunately afflict so many in his profession. The only beer advertisement he liked goes "The one beer to have when you're having more than one." What advertising agency created this slogan for which brand of beer?

A. Schaefer bills itself as "America's oldest lager beer." It's very big in the New York City area, though it closed its Brooklyn plant in 1977 and moved many of its operations to the Lehigh Valley in Pennsylvania. The slogan (and what advertising people refer to as the "campaign" of which it was part) was created by the firm of Batten, Barton, Durstine & Osborne—or BBD&O.

Q. Even though Prohibition became constitutionally mandated in 1920 by the Eighteenth Amendment, in many respects its impact was diluted by a pre-existing de facto prohibition. What was the "prohibition before Prohibition"?

A. There was a war going on in 1917 and one important wartime priority concerns control of vital resources. President Woodrow Wilson badly wanted a wartime food control bill. However, prohibitionists had by this time reached such strength in the country that they were able to tack on amendments that effectively prevented the production of distilled spirits as of September 8, 1917, but—as a compromise—allowed the president discretion as to what might happen to beer and wine. Wilson's response was to severely limit the amount of foodstuffs that were available for beer and wine production and, in any event, to restrict the alcohol content of beer to 2.75 percent by weight. The brewers, of course, were just about powerless to resist. They were almost exclusively German-American, and the Food Control Bill was passed as a war measure to help fight Germany. In any case, by 1917 twenty-five states were officially dry, and in them alcoholic beverages could neither be produced nor consumed.

Q. When Samuel Adams helped to engineer the Boston Tea Party, he was the epitome of patriotism. However, were the same act to occur two centuries later, the valor of the act would undoubtedly be tarnished by charges of "conflict of interest." You see, Sam Adams was a maltster, as was his father before him, and in dumping all that tea into Boston harbor, he was in fact ridding the area of a competitive beverage. What, exactly, is a maltster?

A. Brewing is the process whereby malt is steeped with water and boiled and mixed with yeast and then fermented. Malt is the source of sugars, which the yeast turns into alcohol and carbon dioxide. Malt itself can be derived from many grains, though barley has proved to be the most popular over the years. The maltster supervises the process of malting, whereby the grain is started on its germination process and then, at the critical time, heated to stop germination before the young sprouts use up all the crucial nutrients and enzymes as the young seeds grow. It is the intensity and duration of this heating that determines whether the malt will come out lighter or darker. The darker malts are used for making stout and porter; the lighter, for ales and lighter beers.

Q. Rheingold Breweries of Brooklyn, New York, have produced a number of beers over the years—but its most highly publicized product was the Miss Rheingold contest, which ran from 1940 to 1965. Who was the first Miss Rheingold?

A. All of the Miss Rheingolds—except for the first and last—were selected on the basis of popular vote, via ballots put into boxes wherever Rheingold was sold. The first and last were

selected by the company, the first being Jinx Falkenburg—
who went to star as the female lead in the famous "Tex and
Jinx" radio show—and the last was Sharon Vaughn.

Q.   "Going under a heavy shade tree, I felt the beer come
up, not into my throat, but into my eyes. The day sparkled
painfully, seeming to shake on some kind of axis, and through
this a leaf fell, touched with unusual color at the edges. It was
the first time I had realized that autumn was close." With
these words, Ed Gentry describes the stroll to his office from
the suburban bar where he, Lewis, Bobby, and Drew had
just planned an excursion to add excitement to their humdrum
middle-class lives. What was the trip they planned?

A.   The idea was to canoe down the Cahulawassee River before the dam was built and wiped out all the good water and
splendidly isolated scenery. Unfortunately, the men got far
more adventure than they planned. James Dickey's terrifying
novel *Deliverance* (and the movie based on it) depicts four
men cascaded into a horror of sodomy, violence, and death.
Dickey was poet-in-residence at the University of South Car-
olina when he wrote this, his first novel.

Q.   Beer is a reasonably versatile beverage. You can eat it
for food value, drink it for thirst, or quaff it for convivial pleasure, and it has a variety of properties that enhance its value
for external use, too. Thalassa Cruso, who delighted audiences
starting in 1967 with her TV program "Making Things Grow,"
finds beer an indispensable gardener's tool. What is her rec-
ommendation?

A.   Slugs and snails are every gardener's bane, and Mrs.
Cruso thinks beer provides the ideal organic solution to these
persistent pests. She says, "[S]et shallow saucers of beer among
the pots to lure the slugs to drunken death, for slugs will take
beer in preference to the juiciest leaf." You can use a lot of

beer in this fashion, of course, so give the stale stuff to the slugs and save the fresh stuff for yourself.

Q. Whiskey and other ardent spirits are relative newcomers to beverage trade, becoming widespread in America only in the late eighteenth century. Distilled beverages were a sociable and effective means of using up grain from abundant harvests, but alarmed many because of the effects of high alcohol content. Many prominent Americans of the period decried the use of distilled beverages, advocating beer instead. One such was a professor of medicine at the University of Pennsylvania and the only physician to sign the Declaration of Independence. Who was that man?

A. Benjamin Rush, who among other achievements is regarded as the father of American psychiatry, wrote a pamphlet in 1784 entitled "An Inquiry into the Effects of Ardent Spirits upon the Human Body and Mind," in which he approvingly observed that "many of the poor people of Great Britain endure hard labour with no other food than a quart or three pints of beer, with a few pounds of bread a day." Rush was, for a while, surgeon general for the Continental Army during the Revolutionary War. He has also been called, perhaps unjustly, "the Father of the American Temperance Movement."

Q. Much of American history is sometimes depicted as a continuous war between settlers moving inexorably west, and Indians fighting to retain their lands. Depending upon what you read and when it was written, Indians are portrayed as savage beasts, noble innocents, or pathetic victims. One now-operating brewery, however, owes its continuing existence to Sioux appreciation of a brewer's hospitality. What is this brewery?

A. In 1860, August Schell started producing a lager beer in his combination brewery and home in Minnesota. Curious Indians often visited the fledgling and (to them) curious enterprise. They were welcomed by the hospitable Schells with German food and friendliness. The Indians didn't forget. When Chief Little Crow led the Sioux on several weeks of pillaging, burning, and killing in the New Ulm area, the Schell home and brewery were deliberately spared. Today the Schell Gardens and Deer Park, which adjoin the Schell home, are still hospitably open to visitors.

Q. People always love to argue about the alcohol content of various beers. About the only thing you can say for sure is that modern beers have less alcohol than beers of even a few years ago, in part because the tax on alcohol is a major factor in price, and in part because of modern-day obsessions with low-calorie brews. How do American beers compare with Canadian and British brews?

A. Actually, American beer is in the middle, rather than at the bottom. In terms of "alcohol content by weight," American brews average 3.7 percent, while Canadian ale and lagers measure about 4 percent, and British beers measure 3.4 to 3.6 percent. The figures are somewhat higher if the measuring method is defined as "alcohol content by volume."

Q. Which pricey and highly regarded Eastern women's college was endowed by, and named for, a prominent nineteenth-century brewer who pioneered large-scale brewing in the British style?

A. Matthew Vassar started off peddling a barrel of home brew along with butter and eggs from the back of his father's wagon on a market Saturday. His father's ale, beer, and porter enterprise gradually prospered, but was ultimately destroyed by fire. Matthew then started the business anew and was so successful with his Poughkeepsie brew that he was able to withdraw from the enterprise in the 1850s in order to devote his energies to establishing the Academy for Women, which came to be known as Vassar College.

Q. Most of us are familiar with the victimization of women as "witches" in Salem, Massachusetts, and we know that some women were scapegoated for many of society's ills and then tortured or killed. However, what are "beer witches"?

A. Before the various types of yeasts were specifically identified and isolated, and their metabolic habits described by Pasteur and Emil Hansen and their followers, brewing was a notoriously unreliable enterprise. One batch would turn out well and the next one badly. Everyone had his own explanation. In Switzerland, where burghers took their beer quite seriously indeed, bad batches were blamed on the deviltry of beer witches, the last of whom was burned at the stake in 1581.

Q. Scientists have been aware of nitrosamines as potential carcinogens since the early 1970s, though no one has been able to identify any cancer in human beings actually caused by the stuff. In 1978, a Dr. Preussmann tested 158 samples of European beers for nitrosamines, finding measurable amounts in some 70 percent, with a mean concentration of 2.7 PPB (parts per billion) to a maximum of 68 PPB. Obviously, a huge stink ensued. What, if anything, did the brewers do to rectify the problem—if it was a problem?

A. U.S. beers, when sampled, actually contained very small amounts of nitrosamines (ranging from none at all to 3 PPB). A study conducted under the auspices of the U.S. Brewers Association found measurable quantities of nitrosamines in some malt products, but none of significance in any other beer component (including the grains that are used to produce the malt). Attention then focused on the malting (or kilning) process itself, and some of the nitrous gases liberated in the roasting were soon implicated as culprits. Now all malts in this country are produced by methods that prevent nitrosamine buildup. The Food and Drug Administration is in charge of seeing that this is so.

DAY 4 DIET

Three down and nine to go! That's a natural enough way to think about dieting, but probably not the best one. Just take one day at a time. You can do it! Thursday, of course, was named for Thor, the Norse god whose chariot was drawn by a couple of goats named Tooth-Gnasher and Gap-Tooth. Clearly, Thursdays would not be taken seriously were it not for all the lousy things that crowd themselves into this day. The St. Valentine's Day massacre (1929) was a Thursday event, as was the destruction of the *Graf Hindenburg* at Lakehurst, New Jersey, where thirty-six people died (May 6, 1937). The state of Nebraska picked a Thursday (January 16, 1919) to become the thirty-seventh state to ratify Prohibition, thus making the Eighteenth Amendment officially a part of the Constitution. Nice going, Nebraska!

Today will be a piece of cake (low-cal cake though it may be) compared to some Thursdays in the past.

BREAKFAST:

Today we'll get through breakfast with a minimum of fuss. Drink 12 ounces of water first, and take your vitamin and thiamine tablets. Here's the morning menu:

The Menu   **½ Grapefruit (no sugar on top!)**
Coffee or Tea (all you wish)

MIDMORNING:

It's coffee or tea time, friend. If it's still too early to be sociable and you have a few minutes to break your routine, read the morning paper or get a head start on today's Diversion Quiz.

LUNCH:

One way to cut down on food intake is to make yourself work a little for every morsel. That's our approach for this noon. If the effort gets you irritated, throw some curses at the author of this book, but be sure to stick to the diet. Have a full glass of water before attacking your lunch.

The Menu   Chef's Choice Lunch: Steamed
Artichoke
Vinaigrette
Dip

Once a person gets used to eating artichokes, he or she is likely to become a true convert. Artichokes are ideal diet food—tasty, low-calorie, and time-consuming to eat. Find the largest artichoke globe you can, or two medium ones if your grocer's supply is running a bit thin. Cut off the rounded top so that the artichoke will sit flat when upside down. Place in a steamer with an inch or so of water. If you like, you can season the water with a bay leaf, a few peppercorns, and a clove or two of garlic. Steam the artichoke for about 30–40 minutes, or until the leaves pull off easily. If you don't have a steamer, you can place the globes directly in the water for the same length of time. When the artichokes are cooked, drain them and serve. Peel off each leaf, dip the meaty end in a low-calorie vinaigrette or Italian dressing (use a total of four tablespoons maximum), and scrape off the meat with your teeth. Delicious! When you get to the bottom inside where all the needle-like spines are (the "choke"), be sure to scrape them away and discard them before going on to eat the prize, the tasty and tender artichoke bottom.

The Menu   Restaurant Lunch: Steamed Artichoke Lemon Juice Dip

Many restaurants now serve artichokes as an appetizer or vegetable side order, especially establishments that are patronized by people who like to eat surrounded by a bunch of ferns. One or two artichokes can be a filling meal, well within our calorie allotment. The advantage of eating the artichoke in the restaurant is that you don't have to mess around with the cooking; the disadvantage is that you can blow the whole diet if you dip the artichoke leaves in what the restaurant is most likely to supply, which is a dish of melted butter or mayonnaise. When you order the artichoke, be sure to tell the waiter—on pain of loss of tip—*not* to bring you any such caloric extravagance. Instead, ask for lemon wedges or lemon juice. As an alternative, you can ask for vinegar *without any oil*, and use that, or some Worcestershire sauce (maximum 2 tablespoons).

The Menu   Brown Bag Lunch: Artichoke Hearts Low-cal Dressing

This is a good noontime meal to make you feel virtuous. Get your artichoke hearts frozen; they are available in a variety of brands in the frozen foods section of your grocery store. Do *not* substitute the marinated variety in glass jars; they are soaked in oil and very fattening. If you like, you can get one or two packages, so long as the combined total is not more than 24 hearts. Empty the contents into a suitable container, cover with 4 tablespoons of your favorite low-cal dressing (vinaigrette, Italian, blue cheese), and heat in the microwave.

MIDAFTERNOON:

Try out some of the quiz items on your co-workers and see how they do. Drink diet soft drinks, plain soda water, or coffee or tea, as you wish.

SUPPER:

It's Happy Hour time, folks! If you haven't had a beer yet, feel free to indulge now. Remember to have a full 12-ounce glass of water first. Tonight we'll lean toward the exotic. Some folks are not very adventurous when it comes to Asian foods because they are afraid of what they'll find on their plates. The food almost always *tastes* good, mind you, but the idea of the ingredients can occasionally ruin digestion anyway. Consider Jack Scott's experience, as related in his book, *Passport to Adventure*:

> "I have found a place where you can get a *balut* and a beer." Alfredo went to a nearby *Sari Sari*, a store where you can buy anything from a skinned lamb's head to a pineapple skirt, and got two cold bottles of San Miguel. Following his example, I cracked and shelled the egg, salted it from a shaker offered me by the *balut* peddler, and took half in a fast bite, as Alfredo did, washing it down with San Miguel. "It's very good," I said, looking down at the other half of the egg in my hand. Nestled in the white was half a duckling; a little featherless soft-billed head stared back. I had just eaten half an embryo.

Instead of *balut*, we'll stick with familiar ingredients; but tonight in honor of the nation that produces the justly famous San Miguel beer, we'll concentrate on Philippine cuisine.

The Menu   Chef's Choice Dinner: Chicken
Adobo
Green Beans

This is a classic Philippine dish. Do not be frightened off by the amounts of garlic. It is delicious.

CHICKEN ADOBO

2 ounces soy sauce
3 ounces vinegar
6 ounces chicken breast, skinned and boned
½ head garlic (or about 10 garlic cloves)
½ teaspoon peppercorns, cracked
½ teaspoon salt

Put the liquids in a pot with a lid and add the chicken, cubed to bite-size pieces. Peel and chop the garlic and add that with the salt and pepper, too. Simmer, covered, for about 20 minutes, stirring occasionally, then simmer uncovered for about another 10 minutes or until the liquid is reduced by half. Serve hot.

Meanwhile, cook a 10-ounce package of frozen green beans as instructed on the package. Drain well and serve, with plenty of lemon juice, alongside the adobo.

Menu   Restaurant Dinner: Chicken Adobo
Green Veggies or
Salad

Philippine restaurants in this country tend to be rather simple places, with good food at low cost. If you can find one, you'll still have to proceed carefully to avoid busting your diet. Many cooks add pork to the adobo and automatically serve the dish with huge mounds of rice. Be sure to emphasize that you want only the chicken, not the high-fat pork; and be certain that an overgenerous chef doesn't try to compensate for the lack of pork by loading you up with a double or triple serving of chicken. Forgo the rice, and, as usual, make sure your veggies are free of butter and that you substitute lemon juice for salad dressing.

Menu   Brown Bag Dinner: Chinese Frozen
Dinner

Alas, there are no prepared Philippine foods that lend themselves to brown bag meals, at least none that I could find. However, you should be able to do fairly well with other Asian foods and still stay below our 400-calorie limit for dinner. Weight Watchers puts out a decent 15-ounce chicken Oriental-style dinner, and Swanson and Temple both have frozen Chinese dinners in the 11–12-ounce size that are perfectly acceptable.

EVENING:

Relax and enjoy. If you have had only one regular beer or two lights so far, have another now, and settle in with the Diversion Quiz! It's almost Friday!

DAY **4** DIVERSIONS

Q. OK, sports fans. You've seen the ads on TV until they make you nauseated. Bubba Smith tearing a can of Miller apart to get at his brew. Willie Mays, Jerry West, George Blanda, Bobby Hull, and Mario Andretti beckoning you to join the Schaefer Circle of Sports. You may even remember watching Yankee games and hearing Mel Allen drawling, "Make the three-ring sign and ask the man for Ballantine." Now, see if you can identify the sport whose athletes drink more beer than any other.

A. If you are a runner and you want to be like Frank Shorter, you are going to drink a lot of beer. The night before he won the Olympic marathon in 1972, Shorter quaffed a couple of quarts of fine German beer. Many runners follow the same pattern, consuming brew before, after, or even during a competition. With so many events sponsored (and sometimes catered) by Coors, Busch, Miller, Schlitz, Olympia, and the like, it's probably not surprising that a Stanford University study revealed that runners drink twice as much beer as nonrunners. Dr. Tom Bassler, editor of the *American Medical Joggers Association Journal*, claims that he jogs "a six-pack every Sunday."

Q. Usually when we think of the British Isles, we think of full-flavored, well-hopped brews, but it was not always so. Hops were introduced into England in the late fourteenth and early fifteenth centuries by immigrants from Flanders and Holland. The initial reception was not a warm one, neither for the hops nor for the men who brought them to England's shores. On what grounds were they opposed?

A.   You'll love this. Hops were condemned as a "wicked weed," an unnecessary and harmful additive. It was said that true ale contained only water, yeast, and malt. No doubt many people believed this, but another issue was clearly restriction of trade: all these foreign-born, hop-using brewers were taking business from the local boys. In 1484, the mayor and aldermen of the city of London were persuaded to ban the addition of "any hoppes, herbs, or any like thing" to ale. However, by the late fifteenth century, hops were in fairly general use.

Q.   If you love beer and enjoy reading detective novels, you are probably familiar with Nero Wolfe, the formidable creation of Rex Stout. Although Wolfe keeps a well-stocked bar for his clients and guests, he himself drinks mostly beer, and occasionally wine. How does Wolfe signal Fritz, the master of his kitchen, that he wants a beer?

A.   In 1934, Wolfe was consuming 6 quarts of beer a day, though with remarkable self-discipline, he was able to cut down to 5 quarts, or twelve 12-ounce bottles. About half of these were for daylight hours, and half for the evening. He keeps track of his consumption by putting the bottle caps in his desk drawer—or occasionally in his jacket pocket. When he wants a beer, he rings Fritz, signaling his thirst with two shorts and one long. In some of the early books, the signal was simply two buzzes.

Q.   According to the book *Worldly Goods*, Catholic religious orders in the United States run a variety of business enterprises, ranging from jelly making (the Trappists) to ranching (Benedictine "cowboy monks" ride herd on 500 cattle on a

2,300-acre monastic ranch near Aspen, Colorado) to wine making (the Jesuits' Novitiate brand of altar wine) to brandy (the Christian Brothers). However, no religious orders brew beer—at least not currently. A while back, the Huber Brewing Company of Monroe, Wisconsin, commissioned a series of specially designed beer cans commemorating historical American breweries. Number three in the Huber series was reserved for a church-owned brewery. Can you name it?

A.   The cans in the Huber "American Brewers Historical Collection" were all really quite lovely, genuine collector's items. The third in the series paid tribute to the Benedictine Society Brewery. According to the can, "Father Boniface Wimmer, from Bavaria, established the first Benedictine community in America, near Latrobe, Pennsylvania, in 1844. In 1855, the hard-working monks brewed Bavarian style beer for themselves. Because visitors raved about St. Vincent's beer, it was sold by local innkeepers. The Benedictine Society Brewery grew until 1899, when a lcoal prohibition movement removed the beer from the market."

Q.   One important difference between draft and canned (or bottled) beer in the U.S. is that draft beer tends not to be pasteurized, while beer sold in containers for the consumer is generally pasteurized. The reason is that pasteurization kills the living organisms in beer, stopping fermentation, helping to preserve the beer and prolong shelf life. Unfortunately, the process kills some taste along with the microorganisms. So if you want nonpasteurized packaged beer, you have to find the industry mavericks. Which brewers sell packaged nonpasteurized beers?

A.   Ironically, nonpasteurized beer is available only from the nation's largest brewery, Coors, in Golden, Colorado, and some of the nation's smallest breweries, including Anchor Steam in San Francisco and such boutique breweries as Thousand Oaks in Berkeley, California. However, in order to maintain beer quality in the absence of pasteurization, these brewers need an efficient distribution system and constant refrigeration of the beer, unless it is sold promptly after leaving the brewery.

Q. Everyone knows that Guinness is an Irish stout, and it should come as no surprise to learn that 85 percent of Guinness production is consumed in Ireland and the United Kingdom. Of course, the home brewery, founded in 1759, is in Dublin, snug by the river Liffey, but where are Guinness's other six breweries (outside of Ireland and the British Isles)?

A. Guinness is available in 147 countries besides Ireland and the United Kingdom, with the best customers being Nigeria and Malaysia. The company's breweries outside of Dublin are in Ikeja, Nigeria (opened 1963), Kuala Lumpur, Malaysia (1966), Douala, Cameroun (1970), Ghana (1972), Benin, Nigeria, and Jamaica.

Q. If this were about just any bottle, it wouldn't be relevant, but since it's about a beer bottle, the item is perfect for our quiz: "Polly bent over Samuel's hand and he saw down her dress. She knew that he was looking, but she did not start back or spread her hand across the neck of her dress; she raised her head and stared at his eyes. I shall always remember this, he said to himself. In 1933, a girl was pulling at a bottle on the little finger of my left hand while I looked down her dress. It will last longer than all my poems and troubles." Name the poet who wrote the novel from which this was taken. If you are *really* hot, you'll also be able to name the brand name of the beer bottle.

A. The trouble started after Samuel Bennett got off the train in London, went into the restaurant, and said, "Nip of Bass, please, and a ham sandwich." From then on, it was only a

wee while before he had his left fifth finger caught in the empty
Bass bottle. It seems an improbable basis for a novel, but it
hasn't stopped the Dylan Thomas creation, *Adventures in the
Skin Trade*, from being read year after year in English literature classes. It's probably the most popular unfinished novel
ever written (Thomas managed to finish only the first four
chapters), though exactly why this should be so is not clear
to everyone.

Q. Many of us tend to think of Europe as *the* source for
beer, but there obviously is a considerable difference from
one country to another in beer tastes—and thirsts. Which
country has the lowest per capita beer consumption in Western
Europe?

A.   Italy is the lowest, behind such relative beer enthusiasts
as Greece, Spain, and Portugal. Spain is essentially a one-
beer-product country, with San Miguel being *the* Spanish
beer. However, the beer was not brewed in Spain until 1957
and, in fact, originated in the Philippines, where it has been
produced since 1890. This is a relatively rare example of a so-
called underdeveloped country exporting its highly refined
and successful technology to a European country.

Q.   Ever hear of an Elsinore beer? There is an Elsinore
Brewery, located in Wiibroe, Denmark (which produces,
among other labels, a beer called Hamlet), but the fictional
Canadian Elsinore brand (the unlikely focus of an unlikely 1983
movie) has achieved wider recognition. As the plot unfolded,
we learned that the evil brewmaster planned to take over the
world by addicting beer drinkers to a drug-laced Elsinore
brew. The brewmaster was simultaneously a psychiatrist and
head of the Canadian National Institute of Mental Health, a
role of such diverse demands that it was played by the great
Swedish actor who starred in such Ingmar Bergman classics

as *Wild Strawberries* and *The Seventh Seal*. What was the title of the beer-based farcical movie, and who played the leading roles?

A. The movie was called *Strange Brew*, and the brewmaster is played by Max Von Sydow. The principal characters are the McKenzie brothers (played by Dave Thomas and Rick Moranis), who find a mouse in a bottle of beer and set off for the brewery for appropriate compensation. On the way, we are introduced to a beer-guzzling dog named Hosehead. There are, of course, many jokes and gags about what beer can do to people when taken in mega-quantities (ever hear of whiplash from belching?). Ultimately, Bob McKenzie is saved from drowning in a beer storage tank only by his unquenchable thirst. It's that kind of movie.

Q. Many people who ought to know consider M. F. K. Fisher to be our greatest contemporary food writer. In addition to providing a lot of scholarly and technical information in a highly readable fashion, she is first a highly appealing human being, someone with whom to sit and eat and drink. In one of her early books, *Serve It Forth*, she came up with the following paragraph: "But Englishmen, even then [the fourteenth century] drank ale with greater ease, and used it, moreover, in many of their dishes. They soured it in the sun for vinegar; they sacked fish in it as a preservative, and put it in many sauces. Best of all, they quaffed cock-ale, a special brew in which one lusty rooster had ended his days and lain for many more." What? She must be putting us on! Any guesses on how to make ale with a rooster?

A. For the recipe, Fisher must reprint from an ancient text: "To make cock ale, take ten gallons of ale and a large cock, the older the better. Parboil the cock, flea him, and stamp him in a stone mortar until his bones are broken. You must craw and gut him when you flea him. Put him into two quarts of sack, and put to it 3 pounds of raisins, of the sun stoned, some blades of mace, and a few cloves. Put all these in a canvas bag, and a little while before you find the ale has done working, put the ale and bag together in a vessel. In a week or 9 days time, bottle it up . . . and leave the same to ripen as other ale."

Q. In 1874, the Women's Christian Temperance Union was formed, organized by that driven spinster, Frances Willard. Prohibitionists seemed to be everywhere, and at the U.S. Brewers Association convention that year, the brewers became quite defensive. Their protective posture resulted in an argument that claimed brewing was an economic necessity in the United States, especially necessary since the country was undergoing another of its cyclic depressions. In 1873, guess what proportion alcohol tax revenues accounted for of (a) the entire internal revenue tax and (b) the total income of the United States.

A. According to Stanley Baron, of the entire internal revenue tax, alcohol-related revenues accounted for 55 percent; of the entire income of the United States, alcoholic beverages produced 20 percent. However, 1873 was the peak year for the number of breweries in this country: 4,131. In only two years the number dropped to under 3,000.

Q. We all know about the Organization of Petroleum Exporting Countries (OPEC), yet in truth we tend not to think very much in terms of exports versus imports until supplies related to our own consumption are affected. Now then, where does the United States stand in the world hop trade?

A. For much of the past and certainly for the present, the U.S. is a leading hop-exporting *and* -importing nation. Recently our exports have averaged over 20 million pounds per year, with almost a quarter of our total crop going to such

Latin American countries as Mexico, Brazil, and Peru. We also import over 12 million pounds per year, mostly from West Germany. If you look at an individual brewer such as Guinness, you can see the same sort of pattern: in 1976 they used 20,000 zentners of American hops, 14,000 English, 9,800 Continental European, and 9,800 from other sources. If you want to know what a zentner is, don't bother looking it up in English language books. Remember that hops came to England originally from Germanic countries, and a good German dictionary will tell you that a zentner means a hundredweight, equal roughly to 50 kilograms in metric weight.

Q. In recent years, our social consciousness has developed more fully than in years gone by, and we are aware that indignities at the hands of public officials are visited disproportionately on the poor and the disadvantaged. However, in 1918, the widow of a prominent American brewer returned to this country and was strip-searched by an overzealous Customs Service male physician. Former U.S. Senator Harry B. Hawes called the incident "unexcelled in brutality." Who was the woman?

A. In October 1913, Adolphus Busch died, leaving an estate worth $60,000,000. In 1918, his widow, Lilly, who had been vacationing in Germany when the war began, was finally extricated from Europe after nearly a year of negotiations. She was in her seventies and in poor health. When she arrived in Key West with a nurse and a companion, all three women were strip-searched for concealed messages from the enemy by a male Customs Service physician, reportedly acting on the basis of a spy phobia. On Mrs. Busch he found a newspaper clipping of a patriotic poem, a receipt for $100,000 she had given the American Red Cross, and a photograph of her husband's grave. The U.S. attorney general apologized personally to the Busch family.

Q. "The Sudan is a useless possession, ever was and ever will be. Larger than Germany, France, and Spain together, and mostly barren, it cannot be governed except by a dictator who may be good or bad," wrote General Charles G. Gordon once when he was stuck in Khartoum. That may well be, but the Sudan produces three-fourths of the world's supply of gum arabic. What the hell is gum arabic, and what does it have to do with beer?

A. One gets gum arabic by draining amber-colored resin from the *Acacia senegal*, a scraggly African tree that manages to grow in driest steppe or wettest desert. When the resin dries into irregular lumps, it is collected into gunnysacks, carried to market, and ultimately exported for hard currency. Brewers sometimes add it to beer, as a demulcent, to lower surface tension, to help create the foam most of us enjoy so much. Gumdrop lovers can thank gum arabic for chewiness. It also finds its way into hair sprays, cosmetics, adhesives, explosives, and fertilizers.

Q. None of us like to waste money. Suppose you have some guests over. You of course offer them some beer; and they, knowing you serve good stuff, accept. However, because of poor parental training or perhaps because of some distraction or just plain wastefulness, the louts fail to consume their portions. How can you use the stale beer to good purpose in the home cosmetic cabinet?

A. Many people have used beer as a hair treatment—before, during, or after shampooing. Perhaps you don't set your hair, but if you do, here is a recipe that beauty editor Donna Lawson says will add body to your hair and make it more manageable: Add two tablespoons of strained lemon juice to one cup of stale beer. Comb the mixture through your hair after shampooing. (Just hope the policeman has a stuffed nose if you get stopped for speeding!)

DAY 5 DIET

For most of us most of the time, Friday is a half-open gate to freedom, anchored in the workaday week, stretching into the weekend. If you approach this diet day with a gloomy sense of wariness, your mood is certainly understandable. Fridays are famous for assassinations: John F. Kennedy was killed on a Friday (November 22, 1963), and Mohandas Gandhi was likewise Friday—shot by Nathuran Vinayak Godse (January 1, 1948), as was William McKinley, by Leon Czolgosz (September 6, 1901). Still, better days are ahead, and it makes sense to lighten your gloom with a touch of optimism: some good beer awaits you at the end of the day!

BREAKFAST:

If you stuck to the Philippine cuisine last night, you might appreciate something light and sweet for breakfast. Pour the milk over the raspberries (use no added sugar), and launch yourself into the day. Remember to start off with your multivitamin, the thiamine, and twelve ounces of water.

The Menu **Red Raspberries (1 cup, fresh or frozen), unsweetened**
Skim milk (¼ cup)
Coffee or Tea (ad lib)

MIDMORNING:

More coffee or tea, friend. Allow yourself to daydream about the weekend.

LUNCH:

Fridays are great days for fish, both because of Roman Catholic tradition and because a light fish dish usually imparts a sense of readiness and anticipation. Unfortunately, at this point the only thing to anticipate food-wise is another week of dieting, but all your sacrifices are in the service of an ever-nearing goal: the end of the diet . . . accompanied by a skinnier, eating-again you. Be sure to precede your noon meal with 12 ounces of water. Have one of your beers now, if you like—though my own bias would be to save up for the evening.

The Menu   Chef's Choice Lunch: Crab Delish

This is a tasty and filling dish, quite acceptable to most beer drinkers, even if it *does* contain yogurt. You can add other herbs and spices if you wish, or serve as is:

¼ pound fresh, frozen, or canned crab meat, cooked
¼ cup fresh mushrooms, chopped
1–2 celery stalks, chopped
2 green onions, chopped
¼ cup plain yogurt
1 tablespoon capers
1–2 garlic cloves, chopped
6–8 lettuce leaves (romaine, Bibb, or Boston)
Salt and pepper to taste

Combine all ingredients except the lettuce leaves; mix well, and chill for an hour or two. Mold into an attractive shape and serve on top of the lettuce leaves, which of course are to be eaten, as well as to make the dish more attractive.

The Menu   Restaurant Lunch: Gefilte Fish
                                   Horseradish
                                   Sauce

Perhaps your wanderings take you to a Jewish delicatessen from time to time. Don't despair. It is possible to eat well on deli fare and stay within our dietary limits. The solution is to stick to gefilte fish. If the pieces are about the size of a medium potato (approximately 5 ounces), you can have two. If they serve cocktail size (similar in dimensions to a walnut), you can have about twenty. True connoisseurs of such fare like to liberally dose the fish with horseradish sauce, and as long as the horseradish is not cream-style, you can have up to 4 tablespoons. (This will require a fair amount of water to wash it down.) If in doubt, ask for the red (or beet-juice-colored) horseradish, which is well within our calorie limits.

The Menu   Brown Bag Lunch: Gefilte Fish
                                  Horseradish
                                  Sauce

Again, the I-Like-My-Beer Diet provides the brown bagger with the same kinds of goodies that the expense account people get. Gefilte fish comes in cans or jars from Manischewitz, Rokeach, and Mother's brands, and a good general rule is that you can have two potato-size pieces, or about 10–12 ounces. Horseradish sauce is likewise available from multiple purveyors (including Kraft and Borden), and you can have a couple of ounces of the stuff as long as it isn't cream-style and especially if it is red in color. Be prepared to drown the fire in your throat with plenty of water.

MIDAFTERNOON:

If the diet soft drinks are getting to you, here is a welcome change of pace: fill a drinking glass with ice, toss in a few cocktail onions speared on toothpicks, and top off with water. TGIF! You can have as many onions as you wish. They contain only a trace of calories.

SUPPER:

Beer arouses in some men and women the kind of exuberance that is an important factor in the propagation of the species. Be forewarned. This is the weekend, and anything can happen. Tonight, have a Scandinavian brew (there are many good ones), and we'll have a dinner with the same sort of national origin. Jack Scott will set the tone with an excerpt from his travel book *Passport to Adventure*. He is at a Norwegian mining center above the Arctic Circle: "As we got dishes of the savory stew and foaming glasses, Ben Berg's ruddy face beamed. He said, 'I don't know if I've told you the little rule I have in life: Have a little fun *every day*.' Dunking a piece of coarse homemade bread in the stew and chasing it down with the cold beer, he added, '*This* is the fun for today!' "

Of course we'll forgo the homemade bread and instead of the reindeer stew, we're having fish stew, but it's close enough. Be sure to have a 12-ounce glass of water first, and then have your brew.

The Menu Chef's Choice Dinner: Scandinavian Fiskesuppe

This is a filling, one-dish, traditional Scandinavian meal. Variations are endless. This one has less starch and fat and somewhat more spice than many you will come across:

⅔ pound cod or haddock fillets
4–6 whole peppercorns
1 teaspoon parsley, chopped
1 bay leaf
1 tablespoon dill, chopped
1 carrot, sliced in one-inch segments
½ medium onion, sliced
1 cup cauliflower florets
1 teaspoon chives, chopped
½ cup skim milk
¼ teaspoon nutmeg, grated
2 teaspoons lemon juice
Salt and pepper to taste

Put the fish, peppercorns, parsley, bay leaf, dill, and a pinch of salt in a small pot and cover with cold water. Simmer until the fish flakes easily with a fork. Remove and set aside the fish, and reduce the fish stock by simmering until it has reached one-half its original volume. In the meantime, in another pot, put the carrot, onion, cauliflower, chives, and a pinch of salt; add about one-half cup of water, cover, and cook until tender (but not soft). Combine with the reduced fish stock, the fish, and all remaining ingredients; heat until piping hot. Then serve.

The Menu   Restaurant Dinner: Dinner Salad
Soup
Pickled Herring

Scandinavian restaurants can be very tricky for the dieter because while the food often *sounds* low-cal (e.g., fish and salads), it is often surrounded by so much sour cream, oil, and carbohydrates that you can go through three days' allowance of calories in a single meal composed of gravlax, herring in sour cream, and salads mixed with mayonnaise. Therefore, one must proceed carefully. The best bet is therefore to have a small dinner salad seasoned with lemon juice or vinegar, a bowl of soup (not cream of anything), and an appetizer plate of pickled herring.

The Menu   Brown Bag Dinner: Herring
Soup

With just a little effort, you can make this into quite an attractive, as well as tasty, repast. Buy any variety of pickled or kippered (not creamed) herring you wish, in the 4–5-ounce size (King, Oscar, and Vita are widely available brands). For the bonus in appearance, you can spread the fish on a few lettuce leaves instead of eating it from the jar or a plain plate. Filling soups that more or less fit the Scandinavian theme include black bean soup (in a can, from Pepperidge Farm) or leek soup (from the prepared, dried mix by Knorr). You can have an 8-ounce serving of either.

EVENING:

Ideally, you'll spend the evening in some entertaining fashion. If you have been sparing today, you can have your full day's quota of beer over the course of the evening. Try out the Diversion Quiz with friends!

DAY 5 DIVERSIONS

Q. Prohibition is usually viewed as a uniquely American disaster, but one European country also enacted a total prohibition law. What is that country?

A. Finland suffered from total prohibition from 1919 to 1933. All of the northern Scandinavian countries remain fairly straitlaced about alcohol to this day, with rigorous laws about alcohol content of beverages and restrictions concerning availability. Finnish beer is mostly 2.25 percent alcohol by volume, and the breweries are franchised by the state alcohol monopoly. Norway forbids the advertising of beer, except for those of no or low (2.2 percent) alcohol content, so that Ringnes (exported to and advertised in the United States) cannot proclaim its virtues to its own countrymen. In Sweden, temperance-minded regulations govern beer sales. Beer by the glass is supposed to be served only with meals (though this is not always enforced) and package sales of beer tend to be carefully restricted.

Q. Did you ever collect baseball cards? These little items have apparently been around since the 1880s as a purely American phenomenon. They started as promotional items for tobacco companies and then spread to candy and gum products. Ultimately, hundreds of companies were involved in issuing these popular collectibles, including such products as meat, potato chips, bakery items, soft drinks, and fast foods.

However, only one brewer ever issued baseball cards. Name that brewer!

A.   OK, I cheated—sort of. Because baseball cards are largely directed at kids, none of the alcoholic beverage manufacturers ever produced them—though that consideration never slowed down the tobacco companies. However, in 1928, Yuengling—which is now America's oldest brewery, having been operated by the same family since 1829—produced a set of some sixty cards, including such esteemed players as Tris Speaker, Ty Cobb, Carl Mays, and of course Babe Ruth. Because 1928 was a Prohibition year, Yuengling was not at the time producing beer. Instead, they were selling ice cream and the cards were distributed with their ice cream products.

Q.   Everything is more expensive these days. Everyone knows that. However, in the blur of increasing prices, we sometimes forget to discriminate among different products. Using 1967 as a baseline, which of the following items have gone up the most and which the least: beer, roasted coffee, cola drinks (nondiet), gasoline, postage, hospital room charges, and prescription drugs?

A.   Nothing can compare with fuel oil prices. By 1981, they had gone up to a record 707 (the 1967 price level = 100). The price levels on the other items are: coffee 341, hospital rooms 515, cola drinks 299, postage 338, beer 204, and prescription drugs 180. Because of the sharp rise in the cost of sugar as a result of the Cuban sugar embargo of some years ago, we are faced with the bizarre situation that soft drinks often cost as much as or more than many domestic beers.

Q.   You may not care for the games Paul Theroux plays on the way to Patagonia, but you'll like the stakes: "I asked him to give me the capital of Upper Volta. Andy did not know that

Ouagadougou is the capital of Upper Volta. He countered with Nevada. I did not know that Carson City was its capital, and I missed Illinois, too. Andy knew more capital cities than anyone I had ever met, and I pride myself on my knowledge of capitals. He missed New Hampshire (Concord) and Sri Lanka (Colombo), but that was all, apart from Upper Volta. He bought me three beers. I ended up buying six." Now that you know all the easy answers, like the capital of Nevada, for one free beer from your neighbor, what is Carson City's oldest business?

A.   No, it's not prostitution and it's not gambling. Nevada now has no breweries, but in the 1860s —when silver was king—it had at least twenty-one. The oldest of these (and the last one to survive when it folded in 1948) laid claim to being the state's oldest business. The Carson City Brewing Company switched from making steam beer to the more widely popular lager beer in 1910. They brewed Tahoe Beer, whose advertising slogan was "As famous as the Lake." Arnold Millard, who, in addition to being president and general manager of the company for years, was also mayor of Carson City from 1931 to 1939, has told the company's story in *History of the Carson Brewing Company.*

Q.   When his father died in 1759, Henry Thrale inherited the famous Anchor Brewery in Southwark, England, and a tremendous fortune as well. Unfortunately, he had no talent for business at all and proceeded to lose his inheritance. By 1781, at the time of Henry Thrale's death, there was little to protect his widow from bankruptcy, save for the auction of the brewery. Fortunately, the widow was fondly attended by one of the most famous and brilliant men of the era. The details of the auction are recorded in the great man's biography, a work in four volumes which has set a standard (of sorts) for all biographies written since. Who was that man?

A. James Boswell's *The Life of Samuel Johnson* is a tribute not only to the subject, but also to the devotion of the author. On the subject of the brewery auction, Boswell wrote: "When the sale of Thrale's brewery was going forward, Johnson appeared bustling about, with an ink-horn and pen in his buttonhole, like an excise man, and on being asked what he really considered to be the value of the property which was to be disposed of, answered, 'We are not here to sell a parcel of boilers and vats, but the potentiality of growing rich beyond the dreams of avarice.' "

Q. This won't surprise you at all: like so much of what government tries to do with laws and regulations, the noble experiment of Prohibition was hardest on blue-collar workers who ordinarily drank beer. That was in part because bootleggers favored distilled beverages with the highest alcohol content possible, since they were easiest to transport, easiest to hide, and most lucrative per unit volume. It was also true that Prohibition made alcoholic beverages in general more expensive, and that's always hardest on the poor. One temporary solution was "needle beer." What is needle beer?

A. During Prohibition, some breweries managed to keep operating by producing near beer, with no alcohol or some slight amount below the 0.5 percent maximum allowed by law. This near beer was sometimes served in speakeasies, usually being "needled" in front of the customer—i.e., the near beer was injected with alcohol by means of a syringe or similar device. The concoction was not very tasty and did not achieve any persistent popularity.

Q. What cartoon character, a beer drinker and hell raiser, well known via the blesssings of syndication throughout the English-speaking world, inspired a Scandinavian brewery to name a beer after him?

A.   Thor brewery in Northern Jutland, Denmark, produces a beer named Kasket Karl. In Danish, a *kasket* is a flat workman's cap, of the sort worn by a cartoon character better known by his English name, Andy Capp.

Q.   "I don't like beer," she said—and right away the reader knows that the author will find some means of doing away with the poor woman. This particular clue is from the novel *A Savage Place* by Robert E. Parker, one of a series featuring a very modern sort of hard-boiled private eye who makes his home in Boston. The gumshoe has many wonderful qualities, not the least of which is his taste for beer, which seems to grow and flow with each successive book. "Hard to warm up to someone who didn't like beer," he says in *Ceremony,* and who among us would disagree? Our hero spells his name the same way as the English poet who wrote *The Faerie Queene,* one of the great long poems of the English language. Can you name him—and, for extra points, the beer he likes to drink?

A.   His name is Spenser. He is tough, irreverent, witty, unafraid, and a fount of wisdom. "A man who sips beer is untrustworthy," he says in *The Judas Goat.* You never know when a bit of insight like that will come in handy. As for his beer, Spenser definitely favors Amstel (he even drinks it in London instead of trying the local stuff), but he is also a considerable fan of Beck's, Molson, and Heineken. In *The Widening Gyre,* he calls Rolling Rock Extra Pale the "world's best beer." Spenser, however, has what used to be called a catholic taste; he is accepting of a great many fine brews. In the eight books I have read in the series, he can be observed drinking Rolling Rock, Pilsner Urquell, Schlitz, Dos Equis, Carta Blanca, Kirin, Falstaff, Carlsberg, LaBatt 50 Ale, Utica Club Cream Ale, O'Keefe Ale, Coors, Schlitz, Budweiser, Pabst, Miller, Harp, and lots of generic stuff. In one book, he says "I can't usually tell one beer from another," but I simply can't believe that. A rare bit of disingenuousness on his part, I'd say.

Q.   Beer drinkers are inclined to be a charitable bunch, especially when in their cups. It is appropriate, then, that one of Europe's great beers, important in the evolution of beer technology as well as a renowned export product today, is wholly owned by a charitable foundation. What is that beer?

A.   Carlsberg Beer is wholly owned by the Carlsberg Foundation, a perpetual source of support for Danish art and science. *The Little Mermaid*, a statue that for many is the symbol of Copenhagen, was donated to the city by Carl Jacobsen, who, with his father, was the moving force first in the brewery and later in the foundation. When Carlsberg merged with Tuborg, the Carlsberg Foundation retained 51 percent of the stock in the joint enterprise—and all earnings from the Carlsberg segment of the new united breweries continue to be channeled through the foundation.

Q.   The following selection is from a brilliant short novel, deliciously cutting in the British manner, which, among other things, offers a satiric view of the English literary scene. Think of a common British term for beer and you've got half the title: "He published his first novel at the period when men of letters, to show their virility, drank beer and played cricket, and for some years there was seldom a literary eleven in which his name did not figure. This particular school, I hardly know why, has lost its bravery, their books are neglected, and cricketers though they have remained, they find difficulty in placing their articles. Roy ceased playing cricket a good many years ago, and he has developed a fine taste for claret." Name the title, or even the part related to beer.

A.   The title *Cakes and Ale*, is drawn from the personalities and styles of one of the key character's two wives—the first a high-spirited tavern waitress, and the second a very proper tea drinker. The novel contains many scenes from the author Somerset Maugham's Kent boyhood, and a lot of it is clearly autobiographical. Maugham was a physician turned writer, who wrote over a dozen novels (the most well known being *Of Human Bondage*), over a hundred short stories, and many plays and essays.

Q.   The man who wrote this thinks the best restaurant in the world is in Kansas City, Missouri, so everything he writes must clearly be taken in context: "My strategy for eating in London was clear from the start: eat plenty of fried seaweed and dumplings and crispy duck and crab with ginger and dried beef and honey-apples at Chinese restaurants. Go regularly to first-rate Indian restaurants, which are almost as difficult to find in America as fried seaweed. Find some decent pub food or consume two or three hundred pints of ale trying." What book is this excerpt from, and who wrote it?

A.   Calvin Trillin is my favorite food writer, largely because he is primarily a food eater who seems only to write so that he can consume. He has a particular weakness for Chinese food, which is evident here, but also for barbecue, Jewish delicatessen fare, crab dinners, and also, it would appear, for his wife, Alice. The selection is from a book entitled *Alice, Let's Eat*, which is a sequel to an even better book called *American Fried*.

Q.   As a physician, I am used to hearing all sorts of health claims for various medicines, foods, and beverages. Nonetheless, it's always inspiring to see beer come out well in comparison to other foodstuffs. With this background, what effect do you think beer has on teeth?

A.   You're absolutely correct: beer helps prevent cavities, or so report some scientists at Guy's Hospital in London who submersed teeth in a variety of fourteen different solutions for a month and a half. Those soaked in beer came out in perfect condition; those in fruit juices developed cavities.

Q. All beer drinkers love their brews to be "kissed by the hops," though some of us like our kisses longer and wetter than others. The classic hop used for the finest pilsener beers, the Saaz hop, is grown only in Czechoslovakia, and there are some British-style hops that are grown only in Kent in the United Kingdom. Most hops used in U.S. beers are grown commercially in only four states. What are those states?

A. The hop-growing states are Idaho (around Bonners Ferry and in the Boise Valley), Washington (the Yakima Valley), Oregon (the Willamette Valley, around Grants Pass, and in the Ontario area), and California (around the Feather River and the Consumnes River). Hop varieties include the Old World types (Fuggles and Hallertauer), New World varieties (e.g., Talisman and Canadian Red), and some hybrids (Bullion Hop and Brewers Gold).

Q. Before Prohibition, most beer consumed was draught beer (or draft, as we call it now), consumed in saloons. After Repeal, bottled beer became increasingly popular—and on January 24, 1935, canned beer was introduced commerically for the first time. Highest marks to anyone who can name the brewery that took this pioneering step.

A. The beer was introduced in Richmond, Virginia, by the Kreuger Brewing Company of Newark, New Jersey, in a joint venture with the American Can Company. Kreuger has subsequently been taken over by the Narragansett Brewing Company of Rhode Island, which—in turn—was purchased by Falstaff in 1965. Within the year, canned beers were introduced by Pabst, Heilemann, the Berghoff Brewing Company of Fort Wayne, Indiana, and the Bridgeport Brewing

Company of Albany, New York. The beer can has remained a production staple ever since, though it was an early casualty of World War II scarcities.

Q.   History is composed of people, and names reveal history. Yeast is exemplary in that regard. There are two basic types of brewer's yeast, or saccharomyces. The bottom-fermenting (or lager-type) yeast is named after an extremely popular Danish brewing company, which employed a chemist who was the first person to demonstrate that there are different species and strains of yeast. The name of the top-fermenting one (or ale-type yeast) is derived from the same word root as the Spanish name for beer. With those facts in mind, you should be able to make a good guess as to the full name of the two basic yeasts.

A.   *Saccharomyces carlsbergensis* is of course named for Carlsberg, which employed Emil Hansen. *S. cerevisiae* in one or more of its strains is used not only for top-fermenting beers, but also by some bakers.

DAY 6 DIET

Hallelujah! It's the weekend! Though it's the sixth day of your diet and your motivation is suffering from the dwindles, though you may feel mauled by the workweek and by life itself, though this is the day of the week on which 911 human beings committed mass suicide by drinking cyanide-laced Kool-Aid in Jonestown on November 18, 1978 . . . despite all those things, today is Saturday and existence is once again tinged with hope.

Saturdays are hard on diets because, for most people, Saturday is a day away from work, the reward at the end of a hard week—and for people like us, food is always a highly favored part of any reward. It's also easiest to keep one's mind off food when one is busy, and what most of us want to do on the weekend is to relax, to luxuriate in social activities (usually with food as a centerpiece) or in restful nothingness within easy striking distance of the refrigerator.

The trick to survival today is to clear the house of all fattening edibles (hide the cookie jar, empty the refrigerator of tempting leftovers), avoid social events that are crammed with food, and keep yourself well supplied with glasses of water and nonfattening nibbles always at hand.

As an added assist, the Diversion Quiz will be longer today and tomorrow than it has been for the weekdays.

BREAKFAST:

With any luck at all, you'll be able to sleep a bit late this morning. Take your time getting up. Have a long shower. For once, take 20 or 30 minutes and floss your teeth the way your dentist says you should. (Mine says the process should only take 20 or 30 seconds; obviously he thinks he has a sense of humor). Drink your 12 ounces of water, and take your multivitamin and your thiamine tablet.

The Menu   **½ Cantaloupe**
Vegetable Juice with or without hot
sauce (6 ounces),
Coffee or Tea (ad lib)

MIDMORNING:

As in life generally, here you've got to know yourself. If you aren't going to be on your own side, who will be? If you can stay at home and keep away from the kitchen cupboards and fridge, *great!* If not, you might consider getting your somewhat reduced bulk out of the house, away from temptation. Consider working in the yard (keep a thermos of coffee alongside), going fishing (ditto), or shopping at a farmers' market for the greens you will have for lunch.

LUNCH:

Salads and raw veggies have been an acquired taste for me. When I was young, my mother (an otherwise wonderful woman) cooked all zest out of vegetables, and, as a consequence,

I always thought of them as tasteless and mealy. When vegetables are fresh and crisp, however, and served with appealing herbs and dressings, they can be really great. Don't forget your 12 ounces of water.

The Menu   Chef's Choice Lunch: Veggie Salad

One can hardly ask for a more filling meal than this. Clean your plate, and retain a clear conscience. Chase any fugitive morsels—or store any leftovers for a midafternoon snack.

> 3 ounces vinegar
> 1 tablespoon soy sauce
> 1 teaspoon sugar
> 1 teaspoon ginger, chopped fine
> 3 cloves garlic, mashed fine
>   Salt and ground pepper to taste
> 1 large head romaine lettuce
> ½ Bermuda (red) onion, sliced thin
> 1 zucchini, peeled and sliced thin
> 1 tomato, cut in segments
> ½ cup asparagus spears (green part only), cut in segments
> ½ cup green beans, cut in 1½" segments

Combine the vinegar, soy sauce, sugar, garlic, ginger, salt, and ground pepper and allow to sit while you prepare the vegetables. Wash and drain all the veggies. If for some reason you don't like your vegetables absolutely fresh and crisp, you can immerse the asparagus and green beans in a small amount of boiling water (but no longer than 3 minutes) to soften them a bit. Tear up the lettuce into bite-size pieces and place in a bowl. Organize the vegetables attractively on top of the lettuce. Add the dressing and toss just before serving.

The Menu   Restaurant Lunch: Salad Bar

Salad bars used to be uncommon, but now they can be found in an enormous variety of restaurants and even—Heaven help us—in some franchised fast food joints. In fact, if your travels take you to a place that tumbles out burgers and fries at assembly line rates, it is likely that the only safe thing to eat—whether you are on a diet or not—will be from the salad bar. But whether you are in a high-class joint or a more simple establishment, there are some tricks to getting through the salad bar and ending up with a meal of less than 200 calories, which is our lunchtime maximum. Essentially, you can have all the lettuce and green veggies (except avocados) that you can eat. Fill up on tomatoes, onions, fresh mushrooms, sprouts, and hot green peppers. Avoid croutons, eggs, anything marinated in oil (like artichoke hearts), or anything in sugar (like sweet pickles). Forget the usual salad dressings; instead, use plain vinegar, lemon juice, or—for a pleasant change—the juice in which the hot green peppers usually sit. Of course, forgo any bread, butter, or dessert.

The Menu   Brown Bag Lunch: Veggie Nibbles

I hate to think of your having to brown bag it on a Saturday, friend, but sometimes life is like that. If so, stop at your favorite supermarket and pick up a selection of attractive vegetables: carrots, green onions, zucchini (cut them into strips), cucumbers (likewise), celery, cherry tomatoes, and even florets of cauliflower or broccoli if you like. Eat them plain, with lemon juice, or dip them in up to 2 ounces of any diet salad dressing of your choice.

MIDAFTERNOON:

If you are sitting in front of the tube this afternoon, this might be a good time to have one of your two regular beers or one of your three light beers. If you want to wait on that until later, have some water, club soda, or diet soda handy for sipping. Acceptable nibbles include any leftovers from lunch, cocktail onions, or dill pickles—so long as the label on the jar clearly indicates that no sugar has been added.

SUPPER:

Tonight we'll favor the cuisine and beers of Mexico. The first license for brewing beer in North America was issued in Mexico in 1544, so their brewing history is a long and proud one. Diana Kennedy, in her superb cookbook *The Cuisine of Mexico*, gives us an overview:

> Beer is such an appropriate accompaniment to a Mexican meal, and Mexican beers can hold their own against, and more often than not surpass, those brewed in other parts of the world. Two of the more local beers, not widely distributed in the republic, are the canned American-type Tecate made in Baja, California, and Cruz Blanca from Chihuahua. From breweries established in Monterrey as far back as 1890 come the much-exported and well-known Carta Blanca and Bohemia and the dark, rich Noche Buena, which appears only around Christmastime. And one should never pass through Monterrey without drinking a well-chilled stein of draught beer with a meal of *cabrito* or *agujas*. From Orizaba in the State of Veracruz come the light Superior, the slightly heavier Dos XX and the Bock-type Tres-XXX—in both a light and dark version. There is the ubiquitous Corona made in Mexico City and its dark, heavier version, Negro Modelo. In Yucatan to the

southeast there are the justly touted pilsner-type Carta Clara; Montejo, more like a Munich brew; and Leon Negro, a very dark porter-type beer—to mention just a few.

Cabrito is goat, and not handy-dandy for everyone, and *agujas* refers to ribs of beef, which are a bit heavy for diet food. (You can have them next week at this time.) Despite what you might think from viewing the menu at your local tamale parlor, Mexico is a great fish-eating nation—as you might suppose from a nation with so long a coastline on both the Atlantic and Pacific Oceans—and it is to fish selections we will turn for our Saturday night dinner.

The Menu   Chef's Choice Dinner: Red Snapper Veracruz

This is an absolutely wonderful dish: colorful, full-flavored, and filling. There are lots of different versions of this particular recipe, but this one is a particular favorite and quite low-calorie.

½ pound red snapper fillets
2 tablespoons lime juice
Salt and pepper to taste
2 fresh tomatoes, skinned, seeded, chopped
½ medium onion, peeled and chopped
4–5 garlic cloves, peeled and chopped
1 teaspoon oregano
¼ teaspoon basil
2 tablespoons capers
2 tablespoons jalapeno chilies, chopped
1 cup zucchini, sliced thin, lengthwise
½ sweet green pepper, cut in strips
½ sweet red pepper, cut in strips
4 green olives stuffed with pimientos, sliced

Preheat the oven to 350°. Place the fish in an ovenproof dish, sprinkle with one tablespoon lime juice, salt and pepper, and set aside to marinate for an hour or so. In the meantime, put the tomatoes, onion, garlic, oregano, basil, capers, chilies, and remaining lime juice in a small saucepan and cook over a medium flame for 5–10 minutes until the ingredients are thoroughly combined. Pour the sauce over the fish, scatter the zucchini and sweet pepper strips on top, and garnish with the olives. Bake the fish covered for 20 minutes, remove the cover, and then cook another 10 minutes.

The Menu   Restaurant Dinner: Snapper or Ceviche

Dining in a Mexican, Latin American, or Spanish restaurant is fraught with caloric hazards. The vast majority of places will have nothing on the menu that will allow you to get by at our limit of 400 calories or less. However, if you do a careful survey by phone in advance of actually going out to eat, you may be able to find establishments, usually on the moderately fancy side, which have something you can eat. Things to look for are fish dishes prepared with a minimum of oil (such as the snapper Veracruz), ceviche (a delicious marinated fish dish, usually served as an appetizer, but you can order a double serving as an entree), or salads. Avoid all rice and beans, and be wary of rich sauces. Fill up on green veggies, if they have them, and lots of luck!

The Menu   Brown Bag Dinner: Chili Con Carne or Cheese Enchilada or Beef Tacos

It is possible to brown bag Mexican food, but you have to pick and choose. Incredibly, Banquet brand has what it calls a Cookin' Bag (8 ounces) of chili con carne with beans that weighs in at about 300 calories. Patio brand puts out a cheese enchilada package (8 ounces) in the same range. An alternative is to get a package of frozen cocktail taco appetizers; Patio brand, for instance, puts out beef tacos in this category (about 40 calories apiece, so you can have ten of them). With these dishes, you obviously deserve a beer.

EVENING:

Hopefully, you still have a beer left from today's quota. Sit back, relax, and finish your Diversion Quiz.

DAY 6 DIVERSIONS

Q. If you are a beer drinker and you have traveled in Spanish-speaking countries, you probably know at least one word of the language: the word for beer. What is that word and how did it originate?

A. In Spanish, the word for beer is *cerveza*, derived from the Latin *cerevisia*, meaning *gift of Ceres*, goddess of corn. The English word for the beverage is derived from the Latin *bibere*, meaning *to drink*.

Q. Mexican beers certainly have their partisans, and appropriately so. Who is the famous actor of the 1920s and 1930s who waxed eloquent in the following passage? "I stood hat in hand in the sanctified twilight of that spacious and cleanly haven, like a good Catholic would in a cathedral on his return from arid and heathen ports; and, after the proper genuflection, ordered a glass of beer. . . . The beer arrived—draft beer—in a tall, thin, clear crystal of Grecian proportions, with a creamy bead on it. . . . It was heaven. It was liquid manna. It had the frou-frou of ambrosia, the tender unctuousness of a melted pearl. The planets seemed to pause a moment in their circling to breathe a benediction on that Mexican brewer's head. . . . Then the universe went on its wonted way again. Hot Dog! But that *was* a glass of beer!"

A. John Barrymore had just finished a three-week cruise of personal exploration, which finally concluded in Mazatlán, in late January 1926. It was, of course, the middle of Prohibition in the States and, under the circumstances, a certain amount of lyricism is understandable on the part of a thirsty Yankee coming into a legal bar for liquid refreshment. It is also true that Barrymore had a drinking problem (he had sworn off all hard liquor for the duration of his voyage aboard *The Gypsy*), which helps somewhat to explain the extraordinary poetry the beer moved him to enter into his diary.

Q. Fame and achievement can be so elusive, yet so many grasp at it—or if not at the real thing, then at least at the illusion of it. There are many cities that claim to be the drinkingest town in the United States. I've heard the title claimed by individuals from San Francisco, Las Vegas, and Cheyenne, Wyoming, to name just a few. Now then, when it comes to beer, which city do you think deserves the title of thirstiest city in the world?

A. The answer is hard to come by because apparently no one keeps official figures on a city-by-city basis, but the best estimates put the city of Darwin in Australia's Northern Territory at the top of the list. Michael Jackson, in the authoritative *World Guide to Beer*, puts Darwin's annual consumption at 230 liters per person per year. Michael Weiner, author of *The Taster's Guide to Beer*, gives the title to Bamberg, Germany, at 50 gallons (or approximately 190 liters) per person per year. Both figures make all of West Germany and Belgium (at 147 and 143 liters per person, respectively) look remarkably temperate by comparison.

Q. Back in 1980 or 1981, you may have gone to see a movie starring Art Carney as a cranky and opinionated brewmaster, who sold control of his family brewery to a conglomerate— which of course immediately ruined the special taste of the brew and ruined the morale of the workers in the brewery. Given what happened at the real-life brewery where the film was shot, it may have been a case of art anticipating reality. Can you recall the memorable title of the film and—for extra points—the name of the brewery which was the site of the filming?

A. Carney played a character named Charlie Pickett, and the filming was done in Dubuque, Iowa, at the Joseph Pickett and Sons Brewery. After the filming, the brewery was sold to Agri Industries—which was not satisfied with the market performance of the company (by this time renamed the Dubuque Star Brewing Company)—and closed it down in the spring of 1983. The real-life Joe Pickett accused Agri Industries of buying the brewery only to gain control of the eight Mississippi riverfront acres that came with the package. Agri Industries vehemently denied the charge. In any event, Iowa is now without any operating breweries. The name of Carney's movie, for those of you who are sticking with this until the finish, was *Take This Job and Shove It*, the very same name as Johnny Paycheck's hit song (Paycheck also stars and sings in the movie).

Q. If you like Mexican beers, you are probably familiar with the brands Dos Equis ("XX") and Tres Equis ("XXX"). Those names and the symbols from which they are derived may stem from an eighteenth-century method of grading beer. What was that system?

A. The system had nothing to do with quality, but rather with strength, or alcoholic content. "X" was for small or weak or single beer, "XX" was for middle beer (also known as table or ship's beer); and "XXX" was for the strong beer, also known as old beer or double beer.

Q. These days, the economy is on everyone's mind, and I regret to say that in my particular circle of friends, money has almost replaced sex as a favored topic. I am confident that this is only a temporary fascination, but while we're at it, it's useful to remind ourselves that a number of people have made a lot of money making beer. August A. Busch, Jr., is listed in the 1983 version of the Forbes Four Hundred as having a minimum net worth of $400 million. Can you name the other members of the Forbes list with beer-related fortunes?

A. Forbes lists only one other individual who has a brewing fortune in his own right, and many points to anyone who can come up with his name. That would be Paul Kalmanovitz, who today has a controlling interest in Falstaff, Pearl, and General Brewing (e.g., Lucky Lager and Brew 102). His net worth is estimated at $250 million and is all willed to charity. The other brewing fortunes are family fortunes, divided among many individuals. Forbes lists the Uihleins (who used to own Schlitz and divided up some $350 million among 450 family members when the company was sold to Stroh in 1982) and the Coors (with some 100 family members sharing holdings worth an estimated $650 million).

Q. Let's say you are a fan of the Milwaukee Brewers. When anyone says American League champs, no other team even comes to mind. You remember exactly where you were and exactly what you were doing when you heard that home-run slugger Gorman Thomas was being traded by the Brewers to the Cleveland Indians (whoever *they* are). Now, for the 64-dollar question: Which brewing companies are the ones that actually own the Milwaukee Brewers?

A. Sorry, Charlie! The Brewers are brewery-less. When the franchise first went to Milwaukee in 1970 or so, the ownership group included one brewer, Robert Uihlein, Jr., of the Uihlein family, which had owned Schlitz since the 1870s. When he died, he left his shares in the ball club to an estate in which his wife is a primary figure. In the meantime, Schlitz Brewing

Company has been purchased by the Stroh Brewing Company of Detroit. The upshot is that the Milwaukee Brewers are no longer owned by any Milwaukee brewing companies. Instead a group of some seventeen investors (at my last count) is in control.

Q. You can read all you want about space exploration and the astronauts, but the *flavor* of the people involved has never been more accurately portrayed than in the book from which this passage is taken: "The talking and drinking began at beer call, and then the boys would break for dinner and come back afterward and get more wasted and more garrulous, or else more quietly fried, drinking good, cheap PX booze until 2:00 A.M. The night was young! Why not get the cars and go out for a little proficiency run?! More fighter pilots died in automobiles than in airplanes . . . the system itself had long ago said SKOL! and QUITE RIGHT! to the military cycle of Flying and Drinking and Drinking and Driving, as if there were no other way." Who wrote these lines and what was the name of the 1979 best-seller from which they were taken?

A. Of course no one officially encouraged all that drinking and driving. The dominant viewpoint was: "I don't *advise* it, you understand, but it *can* be done. (Provided you have the right stuff, you miserable pudknocker)." And, of course, those test pilots and astronauts who survived all the self-abuse could rightly be said to have had the right stuff. Tom Wolfe's book, *The Right Stuff*, captures it all.

Q. Up until World War II, the beer can was still new enough so that most cans carried printed instructions on how they should be opened with a can punch—or church key, as the implement came to be called. The first beer can that required no separate opener was introduced in 1962. Which beer pioneered this tab-top container?

A.   The tab top was actually developed by Alcoa Aluminum and was introduced by the Pittsburgh Brewing Company with its Iron City beer. A year later (1963), Schlitz followed suit and promoted the tab top with a large advertising campaign. By 1965, 70 percent of cans produced in the competitive brewing industry had some easy-opening top.

Q.   The time is March 17, 1940, but who are the people involved and where does the incident take place? "The cantina owner promptly put his loudest records on the phonograph to force a gaiety into this sad place. But he had Carta Blanca beer and (at the risk of a charge that we had sold our souls to this brewery) we love Carta Blanca beer. . . . The cockroaches in their hordes rushed in to see what was up . . . big, handsome cockroaches with almost human faces. The loud music only made us sadder, and the young men watched us. When we lifted a split of beer to our lips, the eyes of the young men rose with our hands, and even the cockroaches lifted their heads. We couldn't stand it. We ordered beer all around. . . ."

A.   The place is San Lucas in Baja, California, and the personnel are the skipper and crew of the *Western Flyer*, a 76-foot diesel-powered fishing boat chartered by John Steinbeck and his friend, Ed Ricketts, to collect marine invertebrates from the Gulf of California. The day-to-day story of their trip—mixed with some philosophy, ichthyology, and beer-drinking anecdotes—is recounted in *The Log from the Sea of Cortez.*

Q.   John Steinbeck was consistent in his love for beer and also consistent in his love for Mexican beer, but a reader familiar with all his writings might note some variation when it comes to his favorite brand of Mexican beer. Take the following selection, for example:

> "Doc, I'd like you to teach me more of that chess."
> "You still think you can cheat at it, do you?"

"No, I just like to figure it out. I got a case of Bohemia beer from Mexico, all cold."

"Wonderful!" said Doc. "That's the best beer in the Western Hemisphere."

"It's a present," said the Patron.

Name the novel that is the source of this excerpt. (Hint: it was the basis for a highly publicized movie released in 1982.)

A. The hint may have been misleading. The novel is called *Sweet Thursday,* but the movie was called *Cannery Row,* the title of another novel, and was actually a blend of both Steinbeck novels. *Sweet Thursday* probably contains more actual beer drinking than any other novel ever written, and Mexican beer comes in for repeated praise. At one point, after being presented with a six-pack of Bohemia, one character is moved to say, "Now, there's a beer for you. . . . The Mexicans are a great and noble people. The Pyramid of the Sun, and this beer—whole civilizations have produced less."

Q. So many expressions we take for granted are derived from drinking customs in general and beer drinking in particular. For instance, in medieval times, King Edgar of the British Isles decreed that in order to standardize beverage quantities and in the hope of reducing excesses, drinking horns should be marked at intervals by notches or pegs. Instead of restricting drinking, this encouraged competition, the person who could take his opponent "down a peg" most quickly being the winner. Now, to avoid being taken down a peg, tell your companion where the expression "at loggerheads" derived.

A. "At loggerheads" was of much later origin than "down a peg." In American colonial times, a very popular drink was a rum flip, consisting mostly of beer, but with a tot of rum and some sugar. The mixture was stirred with an iron poker (called a loggerhead), heated cherry red in the tavern fireplace. When the mixture began to boil, according to Herbert Asbury in *The*

Great Illusion, the flip was ready to drink: "Properly prepared, rum flip had a slightly bitter, burnt taste, and was very potent. An evening over a bowl of rum flip frequently ended in a brawl, and the loggerheads came in handy to settle disputes. From this came the expression 'at loggerheads.' "

Q. If you were to list the differences between Canadian and American beers, you could find a lot of nits to pick. Most people would say Canada produces a fuller-tasting beer, and the United States tends toward a lighter taste. It's also true that whereas 97 percent of beer consumed in the United States is lager, Canadians drink mostly lager only in the western provinces, and ale in Quebec and Nova Scotia. What would you guess are the differences in packaging between the two nations?

A. Alas, the Canadians go for taste and ecology, and the Yanks opt for convenience and pollution. Many beer connoisseurs agree that beer tastes better in glass bottles than in cans (though in some blind tastings there was no detectable difference). Canadian packaged beer is overwhelmingly sold in bottles (97 percent), while in the United States almost half the beer is sold in cans. The Canadians use a standard 12-ounce returnable bottle, which has an average life span of three years, during which it makes 20–25 trips from brewer to drinker; no litter, either.

Q. Were you a whiz in English literature? If so, you ought to be able to identify the author and perhaps even the book from which the following selection is taken:

> "Did you ever taste beer?"
> "I had a sip of it once," said the small servant.
> "Here's the state of things!" cried Mr. Swiveller. . . . "She never tasted it—it can't be tasted in a sip!"

A.   The author is Charles Dickens, and this particular bit of wisdom is from *The Old Curiosity Shop*. Dickens was a great fan of food and drink, and few wrote about these subjects better than he. I particularly like the description of a pub (to be found in *Barnaby Rudge*) that begins: "All bars are snug places, but the Maypole's was the very snuggest, cosiest, and completest bar, that ever the wit of man devised. Such amazing bottles in old oaken pigeon holes; such gleaming tankards dangling from pegs at about the same inclination as thirsty men would hold them to their lips; such sturdy little Dutch kegs ranged in rows on shelves . . ."

Q.   In 1960, when Gene Fowler died, his pallbearers included such famous people as Jack Dempsey, Red Skelton, Jimmy Durante, and Randolph Hearst. Fowler was among the last of the great newspaper reporters of the Twenties— baudy personalities, quick wits, adventurous souls who made news at the same time they reported it. When Gene was a youngster of 10 or so, he got a job with the Merchants Publishing Company in Denver. "Gene was taken on with the title of printer's devil, but his principal chores were sweeping and running growlers of beer from the Silver Dollar Saloon. Much of the beer was life's blood for printers in the composing room, and Gene was an admirer of these craftsmen all his life. . . ." What on earth is a "growler"?

A.   A growler is any small container such as a can or pitcher, but as it is used in H. Allen Smith's biography of Fowler, it refers to a pail. The paragraph continues: "The question arises: Did the smell of printers ink get into his soul, into his spirit, and send him straight to the newspaper shops and a career in journalism? Hell, no! What he got was his taste for draft beer (he usually took a few swallows out of the tin pails before delivering them to the printers) and a facility for expressing himself in terms that were eloquently profane, deftly lewd, and colorfully carnal." Among other bits of trivia to be picked up in Smith's book is that the favorite hymn of the legendary evangelist Billy Sunday was "The Brewer's Big Horses Can't Run Over Me!"

Q. British pubs have changed a great deal over the past seventy-five years. Wars have had their effect on the licensing laws and the taxation on alcohol. One of the big changes has been the presence of women. At the turn of the century, pubs were all-male establishments, but clearly that's no longer true. Along with women, the provender of the pub has changed: now one can purchase soft drinks and mineral water, and even fruit juices. The beer is different, too. Can you name the biggest change in British beer?

A. Denzil Batchelor answers the question in his book *The English Inn*: "When I was a boy, beer might have been strong or it might have been weak—the one certain thing about it was that it always seemed *flat*. Today beer always seems to be bottled (in fact, only 40 per cent of it is), and to have the brilliant sparkle that women demand in it. You show me a woman drinking draught beer in a saloon bar and I'll show you an impoverished bookmaker: both classes exist, but they have rarity value." Batchelor may be correct, but the sparkle in draft beer is also due to the carbon dioxide that provides the pressure in present-day draft and beer–dispensing systems.

Q. You already know that Prohibition was a creature of the 1920s, instituted after the Eighteenth Amendment was ratified by the thirty-seventh state on January 16, 1919. Enforcement mechanisms were established by the Volstead Act, enacted the same year, though the amendment actually took effect one year from ratification. However, Prohibition first became an issue in a presidential election much earlier than that, with the German-American community and the United States Brewers Association supporting the Republican "wet" and successful candidate. What year was this election and who were the opposing candidates?

A. In 1872, Democrat Horace Greeley ("Go west, young man," crusading New York *Tribune* editor and out-and-out prohibitionist) challenged Ulysses S. Grant, who was running for a second term. Grant was a man with a special fondness for alcoholic beverages though perhaps more for whiskey than beer. Grant's personal business failures and the scandals of his presidency are often attributed to alcoholism. However, his drinking habits clearly didn't interfere with his military prowess. In response to criticism of the man's drinking, Abraham Lincoln is quoted as saying: "Tell me what brand he drinks, and I'll send a barrel to each of my other generals!"

Q. Life's high spots are where you find them. The birth of a child. Filling an inside straight in a big-money poker game. Being present, along with representatives of 209 chapters of the Chili Appreciation Society International, at the first-ever World Series of Chili in Terlingua, Texas. Now then, if you had been there on the awesome day in 1967, you would have seen the judges declare a tie for the title of Champion Chili Chef between the Texas favorite and humorist H. Allen Smith. One of the judges was a Texas beer company executive. Can you name the breweries in Texas?

A. Judges for that chili contest included Floyd Schneider, a Lone Star Brewery executive from San Antonio; David Witts, mayor of Terlingua; and Justice of the Peace Hallie Stillwell of nearby Alpine, Texas (who later turned out to be shirttail kin of humorist Smith). Everyone knows that chili must be consumed with beer and no other beverage, though tequila is occasionally allowed. Several years later, an all-women's event was held at Luchenbach, Texas—the Susan B. Anthony Memorial Cook-In—and Cindi Craig won the title (she specified that Pearl beer must be used in her recipe). Other than

Lone Star and Pearl, Texas hosts the following breweries: Anheuser-Busch, Falstaff, Miller, Schlitz, and Spoetzl (which brews Shiner Texas Special).

Q.   As a physician, I'm always amazed how resourceful patients can be in using medical problems and illnesses to some positive end. Sometimes the benefits that can accrue to people who are "sick" take more time and energy and assume a greater importance than the illness itself. For instance, patients will sometimes ask me to "prescribe" an air conditioner for their allergy problems, or a new mattress for their bad back, or a hot tub for their arthritis, so they can deduct their purchases on their income tax. It's also true that if I prescribe a beer as a nighttime sedative for a hospitalized patient, most insurance companies will pay for it. However, I only recently learned that beer can sometimes be used as an aid for diagnosing diabetes. If you can get your doctor to order a beer for you as a diabetes test, you can try to get your insurance company to pay the tab. If you are a health professional or a chemist, you may be able to figure out how the test works. Any guesses?

A.   This little gem comes from a book published in 1935 called *Successful Brewing*. A scientist named Fritzerlander is quoted as follows:

> "Beer has sometimes been used as an aid in the diagnosis of disease. It can be observed with some people the beer foam immediately disappears and falls flat as they drink it. This phenomenon, often observed, may be explained by the fact that in such cases, the beer comes in contact with substances which *increase the surface tension,* whereby the foam holding capacity is destroyed. Diabetics often exhale *acetone, diacetic acid,* etc. Such powerfully *surface active* substances overpower the relatively weaker foam stabilizers in beer and the foam collapses."

Q.   Listen to Sal Paradise: "We turned sharp left into the smoky lunchroom and went in to music of campo guitars on an American thirties jukebox. Shirt-sleeved Mexican cabdrivers and straw-hatted Mexican hipsters sat at stools, devouring shapeless masses of tortillas, beans, tacos, and what not. We bought three bottles of cold beer—*cerveza* was the name of beer—for about 30 Mexican cents or 10 American cents each. We gazed and gazed at our wonderful Mexican money that went so far, and played with it and looked around and smiled at everyone. . . . We had finally found the magic land at the end of the road, and we never dreamed the extent of the magic." Can you name the book?

A.   "It was a wonderful night. Central City is two miles high; at first you get drunk on the altitude, then you get tired, and there's a fever in your soul. . . . We started off with a few extra-size beers. . . . I let out a yahoo. The night was on!" From the very beginning of *On the Road*, there's an electric energy, a restless movement, and a lot of beer. The novel by Jack Kerouac launched the Beat generation and changed the way a whole era of American youth thought about itself. It was a hit when it was first published in 1957 and remains in print and still influential even today.

Q.   The United States began to become a major industrialized nation in the mid-nineteenth century. Along with the expanded plants, the impersonalization of the factory, the replacement of hand operation by steam power, and the increased danger and dreariness of production line work, various trades began to organize into collective bargaining units, and the first national unions got started after the Civil War. Where was the first labor union for brewery workers located?

A.   Cincinnati was a booming town after the Civil War and, with its larger German population, the home of some two dozen breweries. Workers were paid an average of $1.66 in 1870 for a six-day week that averaged 14–18 hours each day (plus 6–8 hours on Sunday). The first labor union for brewery employees was formed in Cincinnati in 1879 and became embroiled in bitter strikes in 1881, 1882, 1892, and 1902. The Cincinnati Union joined the by-then-formed National Union in 1886, and the National Brewery Union joined Samuel Gompers' A.F. of L. in 1887. By 1890, the workers had managed to achieve a 10½-hour day, with an average day's pay of $2.40.

Q.   Some people believe that Johann Sebastian Bach was the greatest composer of all time. As Peter Schickele says, "At 57, [he] was at the height of his powers, a position he had maintained for over fifty years. . . ." Bach was extremely prolific musically (listening to his complete works could occupy you for weeks), and he was prolific with offspring as well, fathering some twenty children. Many of his sons and his second wife were remarkable musicians in their own right, too. One of his children is the subject of an authoritative biography by Professor Schickele—and on the book's cover is a portrait of this Bach offspring, holding a musical score in his right hand and a foaming tankard of beer in his left. The tankard is slightly tilted and brew is spilling into the man's crotch, the chair, and onto the floor. Who is this splendid Bach?

A.   P.D.Q. Bach was "a man who triumphed over the most staggering obstacle ever placed before a composer: absolute and utter lack of talent. . . . [He] steadfastly ignored handicaps that would have sent other men into teaching or government, resulting in a body of works that is without parallel." There are many who think that P.D.Q. is a figment of Professor Schickele's fevered imagination, but let the doubters listen to the music (most of it available on Vanguard recordings). I suggest they start with the *Pervertimento*. P.D.Q.'s masterpiece, reportedly commissioned by the Vienna Opera Company (they offered P.D.Q. "ten cases of English ale and a fur-lined chamber pot") was the opera in one unnatural act, *Hansel and Gretel and Ted and Alice.*

Q. You may wish to discuss this item with your barber. It happened to H. Allen Smith in the town of Taxco, Mexico, and he tells about it in a book called *The Pig in the Barber Shop*:

> The barber stepped back and gave me a long look, straight in the face, and then he said, "*Cerveza, Señor?*" This being Spanish I understood, I nodded vigorously and said, "*Sí, sí, por favor.*" He spoke sharply to his wife and she went trotting out of the shop and in a few minutes came back with a cold bottle of Carta Blanca beer. I sipped at this beer all during my haircut and I have often wondered if that barber provides beer every time he works on a Gringo or if he simply decided from my looks that I was a man who would enjoy *cerveza.*

After you have figured out how to get your barber (or hairdresser) to serve you beer, tell me where the expression *gringo* comes from.

A. There are as many different explanations about the origins of the word *gringo* as Mexico has brands of beer. One is that, during the Mexican-American war, our soldiers sang a popular song of the time, "Green Grow the Rushes, O," and the Mexicans began calling the enemy "Green Grows" or "Gringos." Others say the term dates back at least to 1787 in Málaga, Spain, and was a term applied to foreigners whose accent prevented them from speaking Spanish fluently. Another version says that the word is a Mexican corruption of *green coat,* the jacket worn by American soldiers. As long as we're on the topic of language, you'll be fascinated to learn, I'm sure, that in Spanish (which attaches a gender to all objects), beer is feminine but whiskey is masculine.

DAY 7 DIET

Sundays have always seemed to me to be the most American of days. Not that eating, drinking, kicking back, and watching the boob tube all day are unique to our shores. It has more to do with something woven into the fabric of our history that helps our people spend time together, in a relaxed fashion that makes it easier to get to know one another: church suppers and picnics, garage sales and flea markets, rodeos and softball games, and stuff like that. Sundays aren't days for big disasters or big events: they are made of more humble stuff.

Anyhow, today we will concentrate on food from the United States of America. Be of good cheer, friend. We are past the halfway point on the diet and everything from now on will be a cinch compared to what you have already endured.

BREAKFAST:

If you managed to sleep in really late this morning, you may want to consider having a brunch instead of a breakfast. In that event, simply combine your breakfast and lunch. That should keep you filled well into dinner time. Before you do anything else today (you can use the toilet first), step on the scale: if you have followed the diet faithfully, you should already have lost half the total expected, or thereabouts. Next, drink your 12 ounces of water, take your multivitamin and thiamine, and—when you are ready—proceed to breakfast.

The Menu   ¼ Honeydew Melon
Vegetable Juice (6 ounces)
Coffee and Tea as desired

MIDMORNING:

If your city or town has a decent Sunday paper, just going through it should occupy a solid chunk of your morning. Take your time and sip on coffee or tea as you go through the pages.

LUNCH:

The United States has many local cuisines that lend themselves to consumption with beer. One of my favorites is Cajun food from the Louisiana bayou country. If you have access to some, you may want to wash down the following lunch with a Dixie beer or a Jax. Don't forget your glass of water first.

The Menu   Chef's Choice Lunch: Chicken Creole

This dish is a meal in itself.

¼ pound chicken breast, boneless and skinless, cubed
4 ounces tomatoes, peeled
½ onion, peeled and sliced
¼ cup chicken broth
½ green pepper, seeded and chopped
½ cup celery, chopped
4 ounces canned okra
3 garlic cloves, peeled and chopped
1 teaspoon oregano
1 teaspoon celery seed
¼ teaspoon Tabasco sauce
Salt and pepper to taste

Combine all ingredients and seasonings in a covered pot and bring to a boil. Then lower the heat and simmer for 15 minutes. Remove the cover and cook until the sauce thickens to the desired consistency (usually 10–15 minutes), then serve.

The Menu   Restaurant Lunch: Creole Chicken

If you live in Louisiana, you can find this meal anywhere. Many cities and towns now have restaurants that feature Creole cooking; if yours does, you are in luck. Just make sure that you have a serving of reasonable proportions and you'll probably be all right. Of course, avoid bread (including cornbread), rice, and beans—and don't even look at the desserts!

The Menu   Brown Bag Lunch: Chicken Creole

Again, the I-Like-My-Beer Diet comes through for the brown bagger! Simply put out a white tablecloth and pretend you are paying for your repast with a credit card. Your meal is the same as if you were in a restaurant. Weight Watchers puts out a decent chicken Creole frozen dinner (13-ounce size), which at about 250 calories is somewhat over our 200-calorie luncheon limit—but what the heck, it's Sunday, and if you have to Brown Bag it today, we'll allow you a little slack. No cheating on anything else, however.

MIDAFTERNOON:

If you are stuck at home today and you need something to chew on, consider chewing on raw mushrooms. I like them with hot sauce; many people favor lemon juice or vinegar as sauces to dip them in. Either way, feel free to wash them down with a full quota of carbonated water, diet soft drinks, coffee or tea.

SUPPER:

What's more American and more Sunday than a barbecue? As evening comes on, fire up the charcoal and approach your cooking task with appropriate reverence. As James Villas says in his book of celebration, *American Taste:*

> For some strange reason, Carolina barbecue has always been linked with the most God-fearing people—as if the Almighty Himself had sanctioned a bond between man and pig. . . . Down around Wilmington, the most popular to-do is called a "pig-pickin," and they do just that—barbecue a hog and pick the meat off with their fingers while slugging down washtubs of cold beer.

Of course I'm not going to let you pig out on pork, but we will have some food fresh off the grill. Also, you don't get to have washtubs full of beer. Be grateful for what you have got, and try not to worry about what you don't get. Just remember to have your 12-ounce glass of water first.

The Menu   Chef's Choice Dinner: Lamb Kabob
Barbecued
Onion

This meal is a cinch to prepare on a backyard barbecue— or even on a hibachi on a fire escape, if you live in an apartment far removed from lawns and such. The lamb needs to be started first because of greater preparation time, but you should put the onion in the coals 20 minutes before you start cooking the lamb.

¼ pound lamb, lean and boneless
1 ounce lime juice
2 teaspoons soy sauce
1 teaspoon salad oil
2 teaspoons ginger, minced
2 garlic cloves, minced
¼ teaspoon ground pepper
½ small zucchini, cut in ¼" disks
¼ red onion, cut in chunks
¼ red bell pepper, seeded and cut in chunks
¼ green bell pepper, seeded and cut in chunks

Cut the lamb into one-inch cubes and place in a bowl with the lime juice, soy sauce, oil, ginger, garlic and pepper. Mix well and refrigerate, covered, for several hours. Stir the mixture at least once in this interval (if you are not squeamish, use your hands). After the lamb has soaked in the marinade for 2 or 3 hours (or more), remove the lamb from the sauce and thread it on skewers, alternating with the various vegetables. Put skewers on a grill 5 or 6 inches above the hot coals, turning frequently to cook evenly and to your taste (about 8–12 minutes).

The barbecued onion is simplicity itself. Simply peel a medium-sized yellow onion and place it on a piece of aluminum foil with one tablespoon of chili sauce smeared over its surface. Wrap the foil tightly around the onion and bury in the hot coals for 30 minutes. Delicious!

The Menu   Restaurant Dinner: Fish Kabobs

Assuming you have a seafood or fish restaurant near you, some variation on skewered fish shouldn't be too hard to find. If not the kabobs, go with grilled fish, but have the waiter tell the chef to lay off the butter and oil. No potatoes, rice, or bread allowed, but you can permit yourself a small dinner salad.

The Menu   Brown Bag Dinner: Fish Dinner

There's a fair range of frozen fish dinners that fall under our 400-calorie limit, but you have to be careful to steer clear of fish sticks (breaded and deep-fried) and anything that is loaded down with potatoes or heavy sauces. Swanson puts out a 12-ounce fish TV dinner that qualifies, as does Van de Camp. Mrs. Paul actually puts out a frozen fish kabob dinner, but at 600 calories it is out of our range, unless you can trust yourself to stop when you have eaten only two-thirds of the package. Not me—I'm not deserving of such trust! Weight Watchers sometimes has some frozen fish dinners in our range as well. Check the label to make sure they slide under the 400-calorie total.

EVENING:

The weekend is almost over. If you haven't had your quota of beer for the day, now is the time to drink up. In any event, don't neglect the Diversion Quiz. Remember: the weekend is the hardest for most dieters, so from here on out, everything will be downhill!

DAY 7 DIVERSIONS

Q. I'm privileged to know a fair number of musicians; and while they love their spouses as much as one can expect from ordinary human beings, their real love affairs are usually with their musical instruments. Which well-known, gravel-voiced American singer and guitar player is described in the following passage, purchasing his first guitar?

> One Saturday afternoon he went down to a music store in Landsberg, where he found a new guitar for twenty deutschemarks. He counted out the money—about 5 U.S. dollars—and walked out into a snowstorm. First he stopped at a tavern down the street and fortified himself with a few steins of German beer, which he had learned to like. "Then I walked back four miles to the base, me and my beer and my guitar in the snow. I had drunk enough beer to keep me from freezing. . . . They said I looked like a snowman when I walked through the gate."

A. When Johnny Cash enlisted in the U.S. Air Force in 1950, the only real work he had had was in an oleomargarine factory. He listed his usual occupation as "butter-maker." After basic training and then additional instruction as a communications specialist (i.e., radio operator), he was sent to his new outfit in Landsberg, Germany. In his biography, *Winners Got Scars, Too,* Cash says, "I got to where I loved that beer in Germany." It was here also that he learned his first guitar chords.

Q. The time is 1970. The place is the Hazeltine National Golf Club, scene of the U.S. Open, and we're in the locker room. "Every contestant's full name is stamped in green or orange plastic tape on his assigned locker. The lockers fan out from a small social area of thick tables and captain's chairs situated before a bar. Two white-jacketed attendants stand behind the bar doing little more than eavesdropping throughout the tournament, for there is no hard stuff available and the Hamm's and Michelob beer dispensers are self-serving." Dudley Wysong sips a Michelob and Sam Sneed, Arnold Palmer, and Frank Beard all have their beers, too. What do you suppose is the conversation in the background?

A. If there was any mention of sex or the merits of the beer, Larry Sheehan didn't record it in his *Golf Digest* article titled "The Locker Room":

> Wednesday the atmosphere is subdued, uncompetitive. Business is a bigger topic than the game. The locker room is an office. "Invest in land, baby," says one young pro to another. "Buy you some land, baby." Another pro is straddling a bench in one secluded recess of the locker room, listening to a fashionably-suited player's agent, also straddling the bench, explain what he can do for the pro. The agent's attaché case sits open on the floor, bulging with airline tickets, itineraries, endorsement deals, and pills. . . . In the room, within earshot, are men with tens of thousands of dollars worth of apparel and equipment endorsements, spots in TV commercials, and the rest.

Q. "In Bridgeport's early days, the people grew cabbage on vacant land in their yards, and it was known for a time as the 'cabbage patch.' . . . It was a community that drank out of the beer pail and ate out of the lunch bucket. The men worked hard in the stockyards, nearby factories, breweries and construction sites. It was a union neighborhood. They bought small frame homes or rented flats. It had as many Catholic schools as public schools, and the enrollment at the parochial schools was bigger."

This is an excerpt from a book about a legendary American political boss of the mid-twentieth century. Who was he and in what city will you find the Bridgeport neighborhood?

A. The selection is from Mike Royko's book *Boss*, an immensely readable biography of Richard Daley and the city he controlled so firmly, Chicago. When Daley was born in 1902, Chicago boasted some fifty breweries, but over the years Chicago's thirst succumbed to the onslaught from the aggressive Milwaukee breweries just a short distance to the north. By the early 1970s, when Royko's book was published, Chicago's only remaining brewery was the Peter Hand Brewing Company, which itself was bought out by the Huber Brewing Company of Monroe, Wisconsin, in 1980 or so.

Q. I remember when I entered college in the late 1950s; the University of Wisconsin had a reputation for being a very special place, because on that campus one could buy beer in the student union. Whether it was the only such place, I don't know; but certainly my friends and I thought of it as such. Now, how many colleges and universities would you guess allow the sale of beer on campus?

A. Based upon the latest information I could find, 474 colleges and universities allow the sale of beer on campus. Eighteen states set the legal age for purchase at 18 years, twelve at 19 years, seven at 20 years, and the rest at 21 years. Some colleges, such as Bowdoin, Boston College, and Radcliffe, do not allow beer to be sold on campus, but allow it to be consumed by students of legal age. Many colleges now have student union taverns, some of them even called rathskellers (e.g., Bridgewater State College, Cornell University, Northeastern University, to name a few).

Q. It's always fun to watch two bullies get into a fight with one another, especially when all the little fellows can sit on the sidelines out of the way. It isn't fair to characterize either Miller Brewing Company or Anheuser-Busch (AB) as a bully, but it is true that in their jousting for market dominance, a lot of small and regional breweries have gotten squeezed out of existence. In February of 1979, Miller filed a suit with the Federal Trade Commission seeking to stop AB from using the words "natural" and "naturally" in its advertisements, maintaining that brewing was an industrial, rather than a natural, process. Among other things, Miller charged that AB's famous "beechwood aging" for Budweiser beer consisted of dumping chemically treated lumber into glass-lined or stainless steel beer-storage tanks. What happened to the FTC complaint?

A. Who knows? AB says the FTC took no action and so apparently the FTC found no merit in the Miller complaint. Miller says that they have not yet been advised of any official action by the FTC. Somehow, it seems, the FTC managed to wriggle out from the middle of this ongoing squabble between the two brewing giants. According to *Science* magazine, AB had likewise filed an FTC complaint in 1977, charging that Miller was deceiving the public by packaging its Löwenbräu beer in containers that were identical with those used when the beer was actually made in Germany. The American Löwenbräu was an inferior product, charged AB, and the American public should not be tricked into thinking it was the authentic German brew. The FTC declined to get involved that time as well, but Miller modified its advertising to reveal that Löwenbräu was now American-made.

Q. Some people called it the cobalt crisis of 1966. It was that year when a new and bizarre disease started afflicting the hearts of heavy beer drinkers in Omaha, Nebraska; Quebec City, Canada; Minneapolis, Minnesota; and Belgium. After some twenty to sixty people died (the figures vary), the deaths were traced to cobalt in beer. The U.S. Brewers Association took a leadership role in the situation, and all brewers in the United States signed affidavits saying they would discontinue the use of cobalt in beer within 72 hours (all of this some seven weeks before the FDA made a pronouncement on the matter). But what was the cobalt doing in the beer in the first place, and why didn't the same kind of cobalt heart disease (or cardiomyopathy) afflict metalworkers who were around cobalt all the time?

A.   Most beer drinkers like to see some foam on their favorite brew. Unfortunately, synthetic detergents introduced in the 1960s had anti-foam properties; and even with extensive rinsing, beer in saloon beer glasses remained aesthetically undesirable for many beer drinkers. A Danish firm then pioneered a method for adding cobalt chloride to beer, with the result that the foam was restored and stabilized. The cobalt caused no problems in animal experiments and in fact caused no problems with many millions of people who drank some cobalt-containing beer. Between 1964 and 1966, some 20–25 percent of beer sold in the United States had added cobalt. The disease afflicted only those who drank enormous amounts of beer, essentially alcoholics who were also undernourished. The authoritative *American Journal of Medicine* linked the heart's cobalt sensitivity to a diet deficient in protein, vitamins (especially thiamine), and zinc.

Q.   Any institution as large and complex as the United States military inevitably has to suffer from some internal inconsistencies. Take the military view of alcohol and alcoholism. Some studies suggest that 37 percent of navy enlisted men and 18 percent of officers suffer from "serious" or "critical" drinking problems. At the same time, the government subsidizes booze to servicemen to the tune of $16 million per year through its PX system where—tax-free and transportation-cost-free—

booze may be available at one-third of the U.S. retail price and up to one-fifth of the prevailing community price at military bases in, e.g., Britain. In part, this extraordinary giveaway may be due, in my opinion, to continuing guilt in the command structure about Order 99. What was Order 99?

A.   In 1914, Secretary of the Navy Josephus Daniels, in response to pressure from temperance groups, issued his famous Order 99, directing that all alcoholic beverages be removed from navy ships. It had been some time, even before then, since enlisted men had been permitted to have booze on ships, but officers were permitted to do so until 1914. A century or more ago, seamen were given daily grog rations, and British swabbies traditionally counted on their daily ale allotment until prohibitionist pressures affected them, too. When I was in the service, however, there were always two places where one could find "exposure rations" on board ship: sick bay (under the medical officer's supervision) and the captain's cabin. All this led to a certain disrespect for regulations, but it was in service of one-half of Admiral "Bull" Halsey's famous dictum: "I never trust a fighting man who doesn't smoke or drink." Recently, the Navy has agreed to allow a total of two cans of beer per man after 45 days at sea.

Q.   At some time or other in a person's development, it's wonderful to have a tavern that you frequent, a home away from home where you are recognized and feel welcome. This was such a place to a young troubadour: "Joe McDonagh was the keeper of a saloon at Broadway at One Hundred Twenty-Fifth Street. . . . He had come to America, this Irish intellectual, and forced to make a living, he had taken up carpentry. At the repeal of prohibition, he started a saloon. Of all the people who should not have been a saloon keeper, Joe McDonagh was the first. Yet it was a delight for those who appreciated him to be served a beer by Joe and then discuss Shakespeare, Beethoven, or James Joyce." The young singer who recorded these words was later to achieve considerable success on the stage and in the movies, most spectacularly in the role of Big Daddy in *Cat on a Hot Tin Roof*. What is his name?

A. In his autobiography, *Wayfaring Stranger*, Burl Ives describes his warm acquaintance with beer and the singular characters he met in Joe's bar and, even earlier, on the road and in hobo jungles, during his youthful travels as a wandering minstrel. "I sang and we drank, a song and a beer, a song and a beer. . . ." He approaches his music with a reflective humility. Regarding one old tune, he says: "It occurred to me, on thinking of the long existence of this song, that any singer is only a moment in the life of such a great song. . . . A song differs from material works of art in that it only shines when sung. . . . It will shine just as long as there are singers to present its beauty."

Q. Ah, prejudice and stereotypes! They seem to pervade human thought (or the lack of it) and conversation wherever you go. Every nationality, ethnic or religious group, job title, and socioeconomic classification comes in for its share of simplistic labeling and, often, abuse. The German people, in part because of their role in two world wars, are often handy targets. Consider the following: "This nation has arbitrarily stupefied itself for nearly a thousand years: nowhere have the two great European narcotics, alcohol and Christianity, been more wickedly misused. . . . How much moody heaviness, lameness, humidity and dressing-gown mood, how much beer is in German intelligence!"

Which German philosopher can we thank for this observation?

A. Friedrich Wilhelm Nietzsche (1844–1900) was, like many preachers' kids, something of a hell raiser. However, he contributed his mischief by applying his fearsome intelligence to contemporary notions of what was good, true, and beautiful.

Nietzsche led a deservedly lonely life, with neither followers nor disciples, for he rejected everything that others valued (including beer) and espoused notions no one else could stand. He had enemies everywhere, of course, including Germany; and he was labeled a madman, an infidel, a corrupter of morals, a promoter of wars, and a hater of all persons everywhere. Yet as a philosopher, his work endures, and he is studied widely in university departments of philosophy throughout the world.

Q. The book *Old Glory—An American Voyage* describes Britisher Jonathan Raban's attempt to recapture the spirit of his childhood hero, Huckleberry Finn, by traveling alone in a sixteen-foot boat down the Mississippi from Minneapolis to New Orleans. He describes his introduction to Minneapolis on Labor Day, 1979: "The traffic control system of Minneapolis had been switched on specially for my benefit. 'Walk' signs flashed WALK and DON'T WALK to whatever ghosts haven't deserted cities. Blinking filter-arrows sped imaginary columns of automobiles down empty avenues. Somewhere, many streets away, a police car went whooping just for the sake of whooping, like a lonely kid whistling to keep himself company. The sweet stink of a brewery lay leaden in the heat."
What brewery would one find in Minneapolis?

A. In 1979, one would have searched in vain for a brewery in Minneapolis. Either Raban's nose was playing tricks on him, or else the aroma was coming from one of the two breweries across the river in St. Paul, where both Heileman and Olympia had large plants. Minnesota's other breweries are August Schell, in New Ulm, and Cold Spring in a town of the same name, both about 75 miles away from Minneapolis. With these four, Minnesota is one of the top ten brewing states. The others that have as many or more commercial breweries are: Ohio (4); Washington (4); Florida (4); New Jersey (5); New York (5); Texas (7); Wisconsin (8); California (8); and Pennsylvania (12).

Q. "The brewers of America took the foaming promise of television commercial marketing to their hearts," says Lincoln Diamant in his book *Television's Classic Commercials*, "and it has never let them down. . . ." The first beer commercial on television was produced by Hamm's in the early 1950s. Remember the great big cartoon bear cavorting around the "Land of Sky-Blue Waters"? The chorus in the background sang, "Hamm's, the beer refreshing, Hamm's, the beer refreshing, Hamm's!" But what did the bear say?

A. Even the ducks and the geese sang, but the bear said not a word. Over 700 commercials were filmed with the identical sound track, yet no one thought to give the bear a single line of dialogue. Clearly unfair. The commercial was a popular success, but the expansion program it was supposed to promote didn't do quite so well. Hamm's didn't manage to get established on the West Coast in the way it hoped.

Q. During Prohibition (and before, in anticipation of it), several brewers tried duplicating the taste of beer with various nonalcoholic beverages. The most ambitious of the lot was produced by Anheuser-Busch and was called Bevo. It sold fairly well for a while, but ultimately lost a lot of money for its manufacturer. Why was that?

A. Of course, Bevo never tasted quite like the real thing, and that was always a limiting factor. However, its taste underwent the dwindles when Prohibition came along, and that just about finished it off. It seems the product depended on large amounts of brewer's yeast for its flavor, and the yeast was a by-product of the normal beer-brewing process. When the yeast supply literally dried up, the taste changed drastically and much of the market was lost.

Q. If you are an art fan, you are probably familiar with the works of an English painter and engraver, a pictorial dramatist well known in the eighteenth century for directing his satire at the topics of the day. He made his name and his fortune with a series of six plates entitled *The Harlot's Progress*, tracing the rise and fall of a London whore with an unerring eye for human folly, and with an understanding that the principal wage of sin is more sin. Two of his pieces that have been most enduring in terms of their continued popularity are titled *Beer Street* and *Gin Street*.

What is the name of this artist, and what is the moral inherent in this latter pair of engravings?

A. William Hogarth (1697–1764) is widely recognized as one of the world's great satirists. This famous pair of engravings stemmed from the dramatic introduction of gin to the British drinking public and the devastating effect this highly potent beverage had on the many who drank it to excess. In *Gin Street* nearly every character is in a state of misery and destitution. Vice is rampant, and the only prosperous building on the block belongs to the pawnbroker. In contrast, on *Beer Street*, everyone is happy with their foaming tankards, and simultaneously productive and sociable. The legend at the bottom reads: "Beer, happy product of our Isle/ Can sinewy strength impart/ And wearied with fatigue and toil/ Can cheer each manly heart/ . . . And warms each English generous breast/ With liberty and love."

Q. There has been so much talk of late about what is natural amongst the foods we eat and what is not, that we often lose sight of history. From the beginning of recorded time, there is hardly anything more natural than alcohol consumption. In fact, of the cultures that have survived into modern times, only three have existed without an indigenous familiarity with alcohol. Can you name them?

A. According to Berton Roueché in his book *Alcohol, The Neutral Spirit*, the only three cultures to have survived without alcohol are "the environmentally underprivileged polar peoples; the intellectually stunted Australian aborigines; and the comparably lackluster primitives of Tierra del Fuego," at the southernmost tip of South America.

Q. I thought I was pretty savvy about beer consumption in the United States, but when it came to guessing which states had the highest and lowest consumption, I scored pretty poorly. I'll make it a little easier for you. I'll tell you which states have the lowest per capita consumption of malt beverages and then you come up with as many as you can of the top eight beer-drinking states. Using 1982 figures, the states that had the lowest per capita consumption were: Utah (15.6 gallons), Alabama (17.3 gallons), and Arkansas (17.9 gallons).

A. If you guessed many of the most populous states, you made the same error that I did. Wide open spaces are more conducive to beer quaffing than crowded city streets, and the West produces a much larger per capita consumption than does the East—though of course there are occasional exceptions. The heavy beer-drinking states are, in order: Nevada (35.3 gallons), Wisconsin (34.0), New Hampshire (33.7), Montana (31.5), Hawaii (31.3), Texas (31.1), Arizona (30.2), and Wyoming (30.0).

Q. In 1876, the United States held the Centennial Exhibition in Philadelphia. After the brewers were squeezed out of the Agricultural Hall by prohibitionist pressure, they created an elaborate exhibit in a two-story building of their own. Inevitably, the statue over the entrance was that of the patron saint of German brewers, King Gambrinus. Who is Gambrinus?

A. Gambrinus is said by some authors to be a corruption of Jan Primus (or John I), an early ruler of Brabant, one of the flourishing states formed when Charlemagne's empire was broken up in A.D. 806. This worthy is usually shown bearded, grinning and lecherous, sitting astride a barrel, holding a brimming tankard in his hand. Another story describes him as president of the Brussels Guild of Brewers from 1261 to 1294. Truly a character of legendary thirst, Gambrinus is said to have consumed 72 quarts of beer in one sitting. Gambrinus has been honored by the Pittsburgh Brewing Company, which produces a beer named for him. Give it a try if you find it on your dealer's shelf.

Q. In 1960, 20 percent of the nation's beer was brewed in the New York metropolitan area, and half of those 18 million barrels was produced in Brooklyn. That borough has a long and proud brewing heritage, in 1904 boasting forty-four breweries. What are the breweries currently operating in Brooklyn or elsewhere in New York City?

A. When the greater metropolitan area was the brewing center of the New World, many great names had plants located there, including Ruppert, Rheingold, Piel, Ehret, Trommer, Ballantine, Schlitz, and Schaefer. Now, not only is there no brewery left in Brooklyn (Schaefer was the last to close its plant in 1976), there isn't a single brewery in all of New York City. Some blame management wastefulness, some the expense of operating in such an expensive environment, and some the three-month-long beer strike of 1949.

Q. We tend to think of Milwaukee as the beer capital of the United States, but in truth Pennsylvania is, and has been for some time, the state with the most breweries. The first brewery in Pennsylvania was built in 1683 at Pennsbury, Bucks County. Who was the early colonial hero who was responsible for this pioneering step?

A. The same person who founded Pennsylvania, and for whom the state was named, also built its first brewery. William Penn was a great lover of beer, and his own brewery's product was popular at country dances and county fairs. His influence was significant in allowing beer to be sold without the requirement of a license, and this sensible practice was continued in the state until 1847.

Q.   How times change! And, of course, along with the times, values change as well. We tend to think of George Washington as a model of honesty and upright behavior, and presumably he was. Yet behavior that was appropriate in his time would be suspect in ours. On what grounds could Washington have been accused of "buying" his election to the Virginia House of Burgesses?

A.   Washington was one of the richest men in America and also a man with a great fondness for beer. Like many others of his time and station, he maintained a brewery on his estate at Mount Vernon. When he ran for election to the House of Burgesses, he furnished the Frederick County voters with festivities, which included "40 gallons of rum punch, 15 gallons of wine, 30 gallons of strong beer, 10 bowls of punch."

Q.   When I got married the first time, everyone had champagne. It seemed like the thing to do. When I got married the second time, it was obvious I hadn't learned a damn thing, and champagne was again the beverage of the day. Fortunately, since then my taste has matured and I have learned to accept my fondness for beer as a gift of Providence. It was with great joy, then, that I learned about "8-keg weddings." What is the significance of an 8-keg wedding, and where are you most likely to find one?

A.   For the answer to this and many other questions of significance, we have to turn to Frank Tolbert's book *A Bowl of Red*:

> In Texas towns where the majority of the citizens are of Czech descent, a girl's popularity is gauged by the number of kegs of beer served at her after-the-wedding supper. In Praha, Fayette County, and Zabeikville, Bell County, and West,

McLennan County, I talked with many women who'd had "8-Keg Weddings." In Nemicek's sausage and smoked bacon emporium in West, Emil Nors said: "We've had some 10-Keg Weddings." "I remember several 12-Keg Weddings," said Johnny Harnak. "Someday a girl here will have a 14-Keg Wedding, and her name will go down in history."

Q.   In case you are interested in how your taxes are spent, here is an example. The State of Montana Alcohol and Drug Abuse Division helped to fund a study entitled "The Tempo of Country Music and the Rate of Drinking in Bars." The researchers measured the tempo and calculated sips per person per minute for each song. What would you guess were their conclusions? Does fast music make people drink faster or slower?

A.   According to researchers Paul Bach and James Schaefer, "The faster the tempo of the music, the slower people tended to drink." The results were consistent on three different Friday nights in three different bars. They concluded: "Whether slow songs elicit a mood that in turn elicits rapid drinking will have to be tested by further research, such as cantometric analysis." I don't know what cantometric analysis is either, but I think I would rather lower the tax on beer and forget about funding further studies.

Q.   Now nearly 35 percent of all beer drinkers in the U.S. are women. In addition, in some 80 percent of households, it's the woman who buys the beer from the supermarket or liquor store and brings it into the house. As a consequence, brewers have taken the heretofore unprecedented step of gearing beer commercials to women. Who is the first woman to star in a major beer commercial?

A.   In 1981, Anheuser-Busch developed a set of commercials for Natural Light, featuring cover girl Christie Brinkley in a heart-stopping red-and-white-striped bathing suit that somehow managed to leave her thighs exposed up to her elbows. I had many male cardiac patients come in and complain about it. In one commercial, she says, "You don't have to be some macho jock to like Natural Light." Part of the rationale for the new approach is that 50 percent of light beer drinkers are women.

Q.   The United States has only one truly unique beer, and it is brewed in San Francisco. I think of it as a born-again brew, because the Anchor Steam Brewing Company was about to close in 1965 when it was rescued from extinction by Fritz Maytag. At one time, Anchor was the smallest brewery in the United States; but the advent of various boutique breweries in the 1970s (spurred on in part by Maytag's example), combined with considerable growth at Anchor because of the ever-spreading popularity of the beer, makes this no longer so. The term steam beer used to refer to any beer prepared by a certain method, but it is now a registered trademark of the Anchor Brewing Company. What is steam beer and how did it get its name?

A.   Steam beer dates back to the gold rush days of the mid-nineteenth century in California. Because of the absence of refrigeration in those days and the temperate California climate, beer had to be brewed at relatively warm temperatures (60–70°), but steam beer is unique in that it uses a bottom-fermenting or lager-type yeast, which ordinarily ferments at much lower temperatures. If you are a home brewer, you will find this tricky indeed. The accomplishment is made possible by using very shallow panlike fermenting vessels. The result is then krausened (meaning that a small amount of fresh wort is added to the already fermented liquid), which results in a very lively or steamy head. The final product is a full-bodied, well-hopped beverage that requires some getting used to for people brought up on very light lagers. Some of us, however, love the stuff!

DAY 8 DIET

Would you believe it's Monday again already? Sometimes I think about Babe Ruth on Mondays (he died on this day of the week, August 16, 1948). Another thing that happened on a Monday was that Independent presidential candidate John Anderson picked his running mate on August 25, 1980. Remember who that was? John Lucey's name has sort of faded from public consciousness since that campaign (some claim that he achieved obscurity during the campaign), but he had been governor of Wisconsin from 1971 to 1977 and ambassador to Mexico from 1977 to 1979.

Anyhow, this Monday clearly isn't going to be as bad as the first day of our diet. We're practically finished with this ordeal.

BREAKFAST:

Start your day cheerily with a big glass of water, the multivitamin, and thiamine; then sweeten this new week with some berries.

The Menu **Blueberries or Blackberries (1 cup)**
Coffee or Tea, as per usual

MIDMORNING:

Take a decent coffee break and brag to anyone who will listen how much weight you have already lost and what a triumph the rest of the week is going to be. Ask them who Anderson's running mate was in 1980.

LUNCH:

Really getting into gear after the weekend is always a chore. You need something hearty, something of the variety that sustains Eastern European brewery workers when they work in the cool caves and cellars where lager beer must be stored. (Actually, while borscht is usually served hot, it is excellent cold as well.) Remember to drink 12 ounces of water first.

The Menu   Chef's Choice Lunch: Beet Borscht

There are almost as many recipes for borscht as there are Eastern European grandmothers. Some include meat and potatoes and beans, but this one is purer in many respects—and certainly simpler to prepare and with fewer calories as well.

   1 cup beets, washed, peeled, and shredded
   1 cup chicken broth
   1 celery stalk, diced
   1 teaspoon brown sugar
   1 tablespoon lemon juice
   2 tablespoons vinegar
     Salt and pepper to taste
½ medium onion, peeled and sliced

Put the beets, chicken broth, and all the other ingredients (except the onion) in a pot and cook, covered, over moderate heat for about one hour (or even two, if you have the time). Then add the onion and cook for another 10–15 minutes. Serve hot (if you decide to have the soup cool, simply skim off any chicken fat off the top of the broth, either before cooking or after chilling).

The Menu   Restaurant Lunch: Borscht (or other vegetable soup)

If your town is like mine, you probably have at least one place nearby that specializes in soup and salad numbers for lunch. Any bowl of vegetable soup will do—as long as it doesn't have much in the way of starches in it (potatoes, noodles, beans, lentils, barley, and the like). Also, of course, avoid any cream of anything, or any meat soups. If you get a soup that is on the watery side, you can even have a small dinner salad.

The Menu   Brown Bag Lunch: Borscht

There are many brands of borscht available. If you can't find them in your supermarket, look in a German, Polish, or Jewish delicatessen or grocery store. As long as the label does *not* say "egg-enriched," you can have two 8-ounce cups of any of the following brands: Gold's, Manischewitz, Mother's, or Rokeach.

MIDAFTERNOON:

Getting a little tired of diet soda, are we? Don't despair; you haven't much longer to go. If you prefer, drink plain old ice water or some fancy brand of mineral water, with a wedge of lemon or lime in it.

SUPPER:

Ah, the cocktail hour! One of the great pleasures in life is to finish the chores of the day, to relax in a comfortable chair, and to treat yourself to a frosty glass of beer. Before you do, have a 12-ounce glass of water, and then take your time with the beer. As an extra pleasure, you might consider keeping your beer glass in the freezer. Take it out just before serving and you'll have a fine, frosty glass for your brew.

Tonight, we'll sample the excellent beer and cuisine of Japan. John Gunther tells of a visit to, of all things, a Japanese *bierstube* in his book *Twelve Cities*:

> Then, too, the beer halls are worth attention. I went to one called the Sapporo on the Ginza, which calls itself a "health center" as well. A sign outside says in English, "Sanitary Conditions in this Shop," and a price list advertises a sirloin steak for 800 yen ($2.23), an American "Clubhouse Sandwich" for 300 yen (84 cents). Though the menu was in English as well as Japanese, I did not see a single Westerner in this whole large, ambitious crowded establishment. The atmosphere was extremely decorous. Men sat alone with serious expressions, intently silent and drinking beer slowly out of steins as big as those in Munich. Price of a stein: 250 yen, or 70 cents.

He doesn't make it sound very appealing, does he? Instead of going to Tokyo, we'll stay at home and do quite well indeed, thank you.

The Menu   Chef's Choice Dinner: Sushi Salad

While it is possible to make sushi at home, it is a bit tricky and requires a fair amount of instruction and experience to master. If you are already a sushi chef, unleash yourself: sushi makes a great diet meal. For most people, this sushi-style substitute makes an acceptable and tasty substitute. Wash it down with a bottle of Kirin, Asahi, or Sapporo beer.

3 ounces rice vinegar
½ medium carrot, cut in narrow, ribbon strips
2 dashes Tabasco sauce
½ cup small cooked shrimp
1 teaspoon sesame oil
½ cup frozen early peas, thawed
⅔ cup short-grain rice, cooked (about ¼ cup uncooked)
2 green onions, including the green part, cut in 2″-long strips, quartered lengthwise

Put the rice vinegar (available in Oriental food stores or gourmet sections of supermarkets) into a shallow pan and bring to a boil. Add the carrots, stirring rapidly for less than a minute. Drain the carrots, but save the liquid. Add the Tabasco to the liquid and marinate the shrimp in it for 20–30 minutes. Stir the sesame oil into the peas. Prepare the rice as directed on the package for Japanese-style rice. Chill when cooked. Serve the chilled rice in an attractively shaped mound. Sprinkle the peas around the base, put the carrots and green onions on top of the peas, and arrange the shrimp over the rice. If you are a pro, you should be able to polish off every pea and every grain of rice with chopsticks. Take your time.

The Menu   Restaurant Dinner: Sushi

This is another one of those Asian delicacies that many people are reluctant to try because of the sound of the ingredients, but that almost everyone loves, once they have tasted it. If you have a Japanese sushi bar in your vicinity, now is the time to try it out. A typical sushi meal includes 8 to 10 pieces, weighs in at about our limit of 400 calories, and should easily satisfy your now shrunken stomach. If you are new at the game, order a combination plate. Ignore the fact that you are eating raw fish, and you'll be an addict in no time. The beer will make it easier.

The Menu   Brown Bag Dinner: Oriental frozen dinner

Frozen food companies must vary their catalog of dishes from time to time. In the past, I have found both sukiyaki dinners and teriyaki chicken platters that fit within our calorie allowance, but none on my most recent visits to the frozen food department. Maybe you will have better luck. However, two of Stouffer's Lean Cuisine items, either their Oriental scallops (11 ounces) or their Oriental beef (8⅝ ounces), are within our range. Enjoy either one.

EVENING:

If you still have a beer left from today's quota, now is the time for it. Don't forget the Diversion Quiz, if you are tempted to stray toward the kitchen again.

DAY 8 DIVERSIONS

Q. In Japan, 60 percent of the beer market belongs to Kirin, a subgroup of the giant Mitsubishi conglomerate. As the product of one of the world's largest brewers, the brand is familiar to many outside of Japan. But where does the name "Kirin" originate?

A. As with much in the Orient, this story has to do with Confucius. It seems that the Kirin (see the figure on the beer's label), with the horn of a unicorn, the mane of a lion, and the body of a winged horse, is attached romantically in myth to a Chinese woman named En Chou Tsai, who lived some 2,500 years ago. After an embrace that lasted two nights, the Kirin reluctantly departed from his lover. Following a suitable pregnant interval, the woman delivered a child, who was Confucius.

Q. Back in 1880, the man who would soon be world heavyweight champion earned $320 for the year. In those days, most boxing matches were held in taverns and music halls. According to Nat Fleischer's book *John L. Sullivan*: "Bill McGlory's Armoury Hall, on Hester Street, just west of the Bowery, was the toughest joint in town, and Owney Geoghegan's, right on the Bowery, ran it a close second. In those places, fights were billed almost every night, and for the price of a few beers (nickel beers, at that), a sporting man could be reasonably sure of seeing at least one boxer pounded into insensibility." In those days, John L. Sullivan drank nothing stronger than ale; but by the time he defended his championship in the last bare-knuckle championship fight, he was drinking tea laced with whiskey *during the fight*. Who was Sullivan's opponent in that event on July 8, 1889?

A.   He was drinking tea and whiskey all right, but by the 45th round he was throwing it up, too. Some observers claimed Sullivan threw up only the unfamiliar tea, but retained the whiskey. The fight was against Jake Kilrain, and Sullivan won it, after the fight lasted 2 hours and 15 minutes, to an incredible 75 rounds. Bare-knuckle fighting was illegal in Mississippi, where the fight was held, and both combatants ended up with substantial legal problems. With increasing fame, Sullivan's drinking increased considerably, focusing on whiskey and champagne, with an occasional drop of his favorite Bass ale. On March 4, 1905, he abruptly decided to quit drinking after deciding that booze had turned him into a buffoon, a drunken sot. He then became a temperance lecturer, touring the country, supplementing his income speaking on the subject "From Glory, to Gutter, to God."

Q.   As a beer drinker, you know that the standard can or bottle contains 12 ounces (though occasional brands contain somewhat more or less); that many labels, e.g., Budweiser, produce a king-size 16-ounce can; and that others produce a small stubbie at 6 or 7 ounces. Now then, if you order a keg of beer for a picnic or party, how much beer would it contain?

A.   There is some variation here, but you could ordinarily expect a keg to contain 15.5 gallons. That's what's called a large or bar keg, and it's equivalent to 206 12-ounce glasses. The smaller party keg is half the size, 7.75 gallons, or about 100 glasses. If you do much reading about beer, you'll come across a variety of other measures as well. For your information, a barrel generally refers to 36 gallons. A hogshead is a large barrel or cask whose size depends on what it contains: either 54 gallons of beer or 48 gallons of ale. A puncheon is equal to two barrels or 72 gallons. A butt or a pipe is equivalent to 2 beer hogsheads (or 108 gallons), and a tun—the granddaddy of them all—contains 250 gallons.

Q. "The bar belongs to Jack Conder, a former Shanghai municipal policeman and reported to be the best pistol shot there in the old days. His huge fists seem to hold the memory of many a recalcitrant chin. . . . His bar is a meeting place of 'Alcoholics Synonymous'—a group of lesser Hemingway characters, most of them local press correspondents. The initiation ceremony requires the consumption of sixteen San Migs, which is the pro name for the local San Miguel beer—to my taste a very unencouraging brew." This bit of nonsense was written by John F. Kennedy's favorite writer of espionage tales, in this book turned travel scribbler and beverage critic. Who is the man and in what island-city is he drinking?

A. The bar is in Hong Kong, one of the places that warrant inclusion in a book entitled *Ian Fleming's Thrilling Cities.* Fleming, of course, was on surer ground when he wrote the various James Bond adventure stories. The thirteen essays that constitute the book were originally written for the *Sunday Times* and published in 1959 and 1960. Few would agree with Fleming's pallid characterization of San Miguel, but what the heck: it was an all-expenses-paid trip for Fleming, and he is entitled to his opinions, however flawed.

Q. Sir Anthony Glyn makes a number of provocative comments about Englishmen in his book *The Blood of a Britishman.* Of course, beer and drinking come in for their share of attention: "Apart from a common interest in sport, in darts, in a wish for pleasant social company, two things unite the British drinking men in their pubs. . . . One is a connoisseur's knowledge of beer; discussion is expert and prejudiced, though of course never heated, on the merits and de-merits of various draughts and kegs and stouts. . . . The careful landlord does well to look after his beer like an anxious hen, to make sure that it is in the best possible condition, that, if it is draught beer, it has had time to settle." But what is the second subject that unites pub drinkers?

A. The second topic that binds British pub drinkers is the licensing laws, a surprising bit of idiocy to afflict a basically sensible people. The licensing laws originated during World War I in order to keep the workers at home making munitions and suchlike while the boys were fighting overseas. The laws were intended as a temporary measure (where have we heard that before?) under the Defense of the Realm Act, but they persist to this day. The hours vary from one district to another, but all drinking establishments are required to close in the late afternoon and again relatively early in the evening. The result is that in most areas, it is impossible to get a beer at 4:00 in the afternoon or after 11:00 at night.

Q. Last names of people you know often give clues about the occupations of their ancestors, however far removed. "Brewer" and "Brewster" are common enough last names, and refer to persons involved in brewing. What, if any, is the difference in origins of the two names?

A. According to Hackwood, "Brewster is the feminine form of Brewer; and it is significant of brewing being anciently a woman's occupation."

Q. "It is a terrible thing, Mr. Fleming. These people give all their money for opium. Soon they lose their interest in food and then in women. They become sexless, neuter, and waste away. It would be much better if they drank beer, even too much beer, as I believe is sometimes the case in your country." The conversation takes place in Macao, with Ian

Fleming, the listener, taking notes for his book *Thrilling Cities,* and the talker being the gold king of the Orient. This real-life premier citizen of Macao bears an uncanny resemblance to a famous character whose name is the title of one of Fleming's James Bond thrillers. Who is this man?

A. The "enigmatic" Dr. Lobo, in his early seventies in 1959, is described as a "small, thin, Malayan Chinese with a pursed mouth and blank eyes" with a powerfully built secretary and a powerfully built butler, "who looked more like a Judo black belt than a butler." Dr. Lobo, of course, finds Macao a handy place to be, since it has no income tax and no exchange control, and there is complete freedom in importing and exporting foreign currencies and all forms of bullion. Any similarity between Dr. Lobo and Fleming's famous fictional character Dr. No is purely coincidental.

Q. It's strange how some of the brightest people retain an aversion to beer. With a writer, he or she doesn't even have to say it in so many words; it comes out in the description of characters. This excerpt comes from a novel that was on the *New York Times* best-seller list for eighteen weeks in 1982 and 1983. Who is the author and what was the title? "Over his beer in the evening (but he was not a drinking man; don't get her wrong), Beck liked to sing and pull at his face. She didn't know why beer made him tug his skin that way—work it around like a rubber mask, so by bedtime his cheeks had a stretched-out, slackened look. He sang 'Nobody Knows the Trouble I've Seen'—his favorite song."

A. Beck may not seem very attractive for the first nine-tenths of the book, but it's a measure of Anne Tyler's skill that he becomes a likable human being by the time the last page is turned. Of course, he is flawed—as are all the other characters in *Dinner at the Homesick Restaurant*—and, indeed, as are we all. Both the Homesick Restaurant and Anne Tyler are home-based in Baltimore, where Schaefer and Carling have breweries, both of which produce quite tasty brews.

Q. If you are not a country music fan, you may not know this, and then again it may motivate you to go out and buy the record. The name of the song is "Bubbles in My Beer." Key lines are "Scenes from the past rise before me. . . ." and "I'm seeing the past that I've wasted. . . ." and the refrain goes "Just watching the bubbles in my beer." What is the group that made this song famous in country and western circles?

A. The group is Bob Wills and His Texas Playboys, and the album is called *For the Last Time.* It's an upbeat, melodic melodrama, rich with fiddle, bass and piano, just perfect for a tearful two-step. If you look, you'll be able to find it. Other country songs that feature beer include "Somebody Buy This Cowgirl a Beer" (Tanya Tucker), "Colorado Cool-Aid" (Johnny Paycheck), "Big Ol' Brew" (Mel McDaniel), and the loving tribute "I Like Beer" (Tom T. Hall).

Q. Bass ale seems to attract a large and loyal following in the world of arts and letters. Whenever a book or play or piece of artwork picks out an English beer by brand name, the choice will most likely be Bass. For instance, if you were a theatergoer in 1958, you might have seen Laurence Olivier play a Bass-swilling character named Archie in *Variety's* selection of one of the ten best plays of the year. Can you name the play and its author?

A. It was a good year for drama on the New York stage. Top hits included *Look Homeward, Angel, Music Man, West Side Story,* and *Romanoff and Juliet.* John Osborne wrote two of the top ten hits, including *The Entertainer* (the answer to our question, produced by David Merrick and featuring Bass ale) and *Look Back in Anger.* Bass has been situated from the be-

ginning in Burton-on-Trent, and many have attributed the remarkably pleasing quality of its Pale Ale to the high gypsum
content of the Trent waters. Bass is now associated with the
Charrington group, and the combine is one of Britain's largest.

Q.   The most popular alcoholic beverage in Japan is of course
sake. Most people think of sake as a rice wine, and it is true
that sake bears many similarities to wine: it is usually similar
in alcohol content (15–20 percent), in the fuss devoted to its
bouquet, in its general absence of carbonation, and in the
manner in which it is sipped rather than quaffed. Yet the pro-
cedure for making sake more nearly resembles the brewing
of beer. Sake is likewise similar to beer in that it is served
relatively young, as opposed to the aging process desirable
for many wines. *Now. . .* pause for a moment and reread the
paragraph. There is one clear error. Can you spot it?

A.   As it turns out, sake is not the most popular alcoholic
beverage in Japan and hasn't been since 1970 or so. For this
fact, we are indebted to Jack Seward's book *The Japanese*:
"Japan has 3,870 sake breweries that produce 350 million gallons of this derivative of rice annually in 5,000 brands. . . .
Although the production of sake continues to increase, the
Japanese are drinking less of it in comparison to whiskey and
beer. In 1937, sake accounted for 68 per cent of the country's
total liquor consumption, whereas it is now only 30 per cent;
several years ago, beer production and consumption passed
sake for the first time."

Q.   If you are ever browsing through a used bookstore and
you come across a volume entitled *The Intellectual Life,* by
Philip Hamerton (dated 1890), be sure to pick it up. It's a
rare book, much valued in some circles, and potentially worth
a lot of money. It's a series of seventy-one essays, written in
the form of letters to individuals in need of perspective, concerning their position in the cosmos. For example, one is "To

a Muscular Christian," and another is "To a young gentleman of intellectual tastes who, without having any particular lady in view, had expressed, in a general way, his determination to get married." Given the title of Hamerton's book and the focus of his essays, what sort of position do you think he would take on beer in an essay directed "To a student in uncertain health"?

A. Hamerton was on the beer drinker's side, though one might say his compliments were a bit backhanded: "It is not always easy for great brain workers to follow with perfect fidelity the customs of people about them. . . . A good example of this is Kant's intense antipathy to beer. It did not suit him, and he was right in his non-conformity to German usage on this point, but he was mistaken in believing beer to be universally injurious. . . . Notwithstanding Kant's horror of beer, that honest northern drink deserves our friendly recognition. It has quite a peculiar effect on the nervous system, giving a rest and calm which no other drink can procure for it so safely. . . . It is said that beer drinkers are slow, and a little stupid; that they have an ox-like placidity not quite favorable to any brilliant intellectual display. But there are times when this placidity is what the laboring brain most needs. After the agitation of too active thinking, there is safety in a tankard of ale. The wine drinkers are agile, but they are excitable; the beer drinkers are heavy, but in their heaviness there is peace."

Q. So far as I have been able to discover, only one major brewer has been active as an owner in basketball, and that was Ballantine. In the 1968-69 season, Ballantine owned a club and then sold it to a group called Transnational Communications. However, Ballantine apparently couldn't stand being out of the action, so they soon bought the same club back again, this time using an investors' group called Ballantine Investors Funding. What was the name of the NBA team involved?

A. Those were pretty good years for the Boston Celtics. They beat Los Angeles for the NBA title in both 1968 and 1969. Team stars included Bill Russell and John Havlicek. However, Ballantine didn't last as an owner of the Celtics and in 1972 they again sold the club, this time apparently for good.

Q. OK, we're going to talk some trash here—and what could be more symbolic of trash than beer bottles? However, before all those bottles end up as trash, they have the noble function of serving as containers for our favorite beverage. You have noticed, of course, that beer bottles come in three basic colors: brown, green, and clear glass. Which, if any, is best for preserving the taste of the beer?

A. The clear glass shows off the beer to best advantage while it's still in the bottle (as you can tell from all those Miller commercials), but I have yet to find anyone who says clear glass is good for the beer. Light is the major enemy of beer preservation, and it may be that even green glass does not effectively screen out light. When light reaches beer, it causes a photochemical reaction resulting in a stale flavor which some folks call skunkiness. Anyhow, a national beer consumers organization, the Campaign for Authentic Beer, has petitioned brewers to refrain from packaging beer in green bottles, and instead use the more traditional brown. Some folks say that photochemical reaction is most likely to occur when the beer contains a lot of genuine hops, but is unlikely to occur if hop extract is used—so maybe the clear glass doesn't make any difference with the many domestic brews prepared with the extract. Who knows? You pays your money and you takes your choice!

Q. Some things are beyond politics, and I think this is one of them. Up until 1978, it was illegal to make home brew. In that year, a congressman (who shall remain nameless) introduced a bill that would have made home brewing legal, but would simultaneously have required such brewers to register with the federal government (failure to comply could have been punished by one year in jail and a $1,000 fine) and to limit volume on hand to 30 gallons. Amateur winemakers were not burdened by such registration and were allowed to produce up to 200 gallons per year per household. Now, enter our hero to right an obvious wrong. Which senator introduced the bill to provide equal treatment in home production of beer and wine?

A.   California Senator Alan Cranston tacked on an amendment to a bill concerning excise taxes on trucks, buses, tractors and suchlike—and the resulting law made home brewing legal, up to 100 gallons per year for a single adult and up to 200 gallons for a household. In his argument, Cranston pointed to registration as a foolish waste of everybody's time, energy, and money. He also mentioned that while the numerous home brewers currently in production were technically criminals, the Bureau of Alcohol, Tobacco and Firearms had "not made any arrests of small-scale home brewers since Prohibition was repealed."

DAY **9** DIET

Today is Tuesday again, and your diet is wending its way toward its dreary conclusion, now much closer than last week at this time. This Tuesday is therefore brighter than the last one. Tuesdays aren't all bad. It was on a Tuesday that the Twenty-first Amendment was finally ratified, abolishing Prohibition (December 5, 1933), and it was on this day of the week that Canada announced it had helped spirit six U.S. Embassy officials out of Iran during the humiliating and depressing Ayatollah hostage drama (January 29, 1980). Raise your glass in a toast to Canada (not before breakfast, please)!

BREAKFAST:

Up and at 'em, champ. There's less of you to drag out of bed than when you started this damn diet. Don't forget your 12 ounces of water, your multivitamin and your thiamine tablet.

The Menu   **½ Grapefruit, with one maraschino cherry stuck in the middle to brighten your day**
Coffee or Tea, as you like

MIDMORNING:

More coffee or tea. Stay away from any carbohydrates in your vicinity. Lunch is coming soon, and it will be filling.

LUNCH:

Today, we'll have a lunch of French origin. Most people think of France as a wine country, which is true enough, but beer also has its proud place in French history. If you are having beer with lunch, consider a Kronenbourg from France (actually Alsace) or one of the many fine Canadian brews. Don't forget to have 12 ounces of water first.

The Menu   Chef's Choice Lunch: Ratatouille

This is a vegetable stew, very tasty. This particular recipe is my own, but dozens of variations can be found. Most of them are fairly low-cal, but the amount of cooking oil must be watched carefully to keep it within our 200-calorie limit.

   1 teaspoon olive oil
3–4 garlic cloves, chopped
  ½ medium onion, peeled and coarsely chopped
  ½ cup mushrooms, sliced
  1 cup eggplant, peeled and cubed
  1 tomato, peeled, seeded, and cubed
  1 cup zucchini, cut in thick disks
  ¼ green pepper, coarsely chopped
  1 celery stalk (including leaves), chopped
  ½ teaspoon oregano
  ½ teaspoon basil
    Salt and pepper to taste

For best results, use a nonstick saucepan. Heat the oil; add garlic, onions, and mushrooms, and sauté until slightly wilted. Add remaining ingredients and cook over low heat until vegetables are tender but not mushy, stirring occasionally (20–30 minutes). Can be served either hot or chilled.

The Menu   Restaurant Lunch: Ratatouille

Ever try to order a beer in a French restaurant? There's not much chance of success unless a bar is attached to the eatery. However, if you dine out very often, you will inevitably find your way into a Chez Maison or some such, so it's well and good to be prepared. Stick to the ratatouille, and avoid all the dishes with rich cream sauces, pounds of butter, wrapped in puff pastry. The only caloric dangers in the dish are if it is cooked with too much oil or if some rebellious chef decides to toss in some meat or starches.

The Menu   Brown Bag Lunch: Ratatouille

Here's another opportunity for the brown bagger to dine as well as everyone else. Stouffer makes a very tasty 10-ounce version of this dish. It's low-calorie enough (120 calories) that you can also have an apple for dessert (no more than ⅓ pound in weight).

MIDAFTERNOON:

Take time out for some ice water, coffee, tea, or diet soda. Spend some time with the Diversion Quiz if you get restless.

SUPPER:

Tonight we'll turn to the Emerald Isle for our repast, but if you think that means something heavy and fattening, you are mistaken. Eleanor Early, a Washington travel columnist, once wrote of her visit to Ireland that:

> Corned beef and cabbage, which some Americans think is Ireland's national dish, is seldom used. I saw it on a menu only once. But there are trout and smoked salmon, lobsters, prawns from the Irish Sea, oysters with Guinness. In Dublin (site of the Guinness Brewery) no one would eat oysters without a bottle of stout to bring out the flavor. At the National Stud, stallions receive two pints a day, and the grooms get one.

All of which goes to show that we're having oysters for supper today—and why not enjoy them with a Guinness? At 167 calories per 11.4-ounce bottle, Guinness is slightly more fattening than most lagers, but hardly enough to worry about if you are only having one. Guinness is even better fresh, on draught (draft to us Yanks), but the usual draught Guinness is likely to be a pint (16 ounces), which ups the ante a bit. If Guinness is too heavy or bitter for you, consider a Harp lager, a Killian's Irish Red, or one of the many fine Scottish ales. In any event, have your 12 ounces of water first.

The Menu   Chef's Choice Dinner: Fresh Oysters Salad

"He was a bold man that first eat an oyster," said Jonathan Swift, and who could disagree? Yet we no longer have to worry about being first; we *know* what a treat fresh oysters can be. If the oysters are of the smaller, Eastern variety (about 1″ across when lying in the shell), you can have as many as eighteen. If they are the larger, Western or Pacific variety (2″ or more across), you had best settle for only six. Select only those whose shells are tightly closed. To prepare them, run them under cold water to get off any extra dirt, pry open shells, and serve on the half-shell over crushed ice. Traditional accompaniments include cayenne, hot sauce, lemon wedges, ground pepper, or horseradish sauce. Follow this dish at your leisure with a green salad, such as the ones described on the lunch menus on Days 3 or 6.

The Menu Restaurant Dinner: Fresh Oysters
Salad

Most seafood restaurants will be able to accommodate you on this one. Remember to avoid the temptation of bread and butter or oyster crackers, which may find their way onto your table. If the oysters are the small East Coast variety, you can order up to eighteen; if the large Pacific oyster, stop with half a dozen. Take your time and enjoy each bite. Then follow up with a small dinner salad.

The Menu Brown Bag Dinner: Oysters
Fresh Veggies

The best oysters are those fresh out of the shell. There are many brands of canned oysters, but they are not to be recommended. An acceptable substitute, however, is oysters fresh chilled in the jar, stamped with expiration date, available in the seafood section of many supermarkets. For instance, Puget Sound brand sells a 10-ounce jar of medium Pacific oysters. You can't easily serve such delicacies in the half-shell, but any small dish will do. Season with pepper or lemon or whatever sauce you prefer. Complete your meal with a brown bag selection of fresh veggies: e.g., scallions, cherry tomatoes, celery stalks, cucumbers, and the like.

EVENING:

Tonight the pearl in your oyster will be our Diversion Quiz and—if you haven't already sucked up your quota—another beer. Enjoy.

DAY **9** DIVERSIONS

Q. If you, like me, are of the age group that tends to be called middle-aged, and you are asked to think of a tune in which beer is the dominant theme, you will most likely think of the "Beer Barrel Polka," also known as "Roll Out the Barrel." It was originally a Czech number. Which singing group introduced it into the United States?

A. If you said the Andrews Sisters, that's pretty good. They put out a best-selling record in 1939 on the Decca label—78 rpm, of course. However, it was really introduced into the U.S. by Will Glahe and his Musette Orchestra. The original Czech title is "Skoda Lasky" (meaning "Lost Love") and the English words were written by Lew Brown.

Q. Start off with an interest in beer, and you can learn about *anything.* "In taverns of low repute the patrons may sometimes be observed to sprinkle salt into their beer. They do so not because they like salty beer, but because they are amused by the resulting profusion of bubbles." So say Craig Bohren and Gail Brown in an article entitled, "Cloud Physics in a Glass of Beer," which uses a salt shaker and a glass of beer to reveal some basic principles of atmospheric physics. Now why do you suppose that salt causes all the bubbles in beer?

A. If you thought it was because the salt dissolved, resulting in a chemical reaction between the beer and the salt, you were wrong. You can do the same trick with grains of sand, though it tends to make the beer a bit gritty when you drink it. The answer is that beer contains a lot of carbon dioxide (CO_2) at high pressure. As it sits in the glass, the CO_2 escapes from solution slowly in the form of small bubbles. These bubbles don't form randomly, but rather from a number of sites on the bottom and sides of the glass, often on microscopic cracks or even on particles of dirt. Because of surface tension, bubbles need what is called a nucleation site in order to form, something that breaks up the natural cohesion of the solution— which is what the salt crystals provide. If you want to read more about such topics as cloud formation, bubble behavior, and cloud droplet behavior, consult the article.

Q.   Let's talk about something important. Are you up on your saints? November 12 is the saint's day for the man who is patron saint of tavern keepers and drunkards. Can you name him?

A.   St. Martin is the patron saint of dispensers of good cheer. According to *The Book of Days*, he was so modest and unassuming that he "hid in a barn because he didn't want to be made a bishop, but a goose gave his presence away." St. Theodotus (May 18) has been chosen the patron saint of innkeepers, but of course that is a different matter entirely.

Q.   Brewing is truly an ancient art, mentioned in the Egyptian *Book of the Dead* some 5,000 years ago. Beer making was reputedly invented by Osiris, god of the dead and of resurrection, a very important deity during his time. He married his sister, Isis, who became the patroness of brewers and also the goddess of motherhood and fertility. Whatever happened to good old Osiris?

A.   This is more interesting than you might think. According to *Who's Who in Egyptian Mythology*, Osiris was killed by his brother who, after a number of intervening adventures, also dismembered the corpse into fourteen pieces. Eventually "Isis collected all the pieces of her husband except for the penis, which had been devoured by a fish. Isis then constructed a phallus to take the place of her husband's, and a festival was held in its honor." The next time you run out of things to toast while raising glasses with friends, you might think of Osiris and Isis.

Q. According to the *Book of Sports Lists #3,* "A few years ago, the Miller Brewing Company received kudos, and increased sales, for its clever commercials depicting former athletes. As a retaliatory campaign, competitor Anheuser-Busch wooed several of Miller's former jocks over to its product, Natural Light Beer, with the pronouncement that these men switched. 'Taste is why you'll switch,' is the company slogan. Taste, that is, in nice clothes, big cars, and large bank accounts." How many of those athletes, who would rather switch than fight, can you name?

A. The athletes who switched include: Mickey Mantle, Knicks basketball hero Walt Frazier, heavyweight champ Joe Frazier, Washington Redskins quarterback Sonny Jorgenson, hockey star Gordie Howe, Yankee pitcher Catfish Hunter, Dodger manager Tom Lasorda, and Miami Dolphin linebacker Nick Buoniconti.

Q. As a beer drinker, if you come across a book called *Ambrosia and Small Beer,* you would probably pick it up as I did. Whether you would like it or not would depend a lot on your taste in literature. It's a record of correspondence between Edward Marsh and Christopher Hassall, arranged by the latter. Marsh was for twenty-five years the private secretary of Winston Churchill, and for fifty years his friend. When he died at 80, he was still a thoroughly lively personality, with a keen and perceptive mind, and with the British talent for using the pen as a scalpel (or perhaps manicure scissors would be more apt in this case). Christopher Hassall is a much younger man, a good foil for showing off Marsh's wit. The book is full of chatter and gossip, elevated by breeding and famous friends and acquaintances to the level of culture. Now, what is the significance of the words in the title?

A. *Ambrosia* is a term derived from Greek mythology and refers to the food of the gods. By extension, it can be used to denote anything exquisitely delightful, something belonging in heaven and worthy of the gods. Small beer, on the other hand, is the weakest and least tasty of brews, pretty ordinary stuff. Figuratively speaking, the term *small beer* is used to refer to small things and trifling matters. In choosing the title *Ambrosia and Small Beer,* Hassall is telling us that he has included some pretty terrific material, but also a record of some fairly ordinary day-to-day correspondence that he hopes will nonetheless interest us. You will look in vain for anything written about the beverage beer.

Q. It was just after the turn of the century and the following scene is taken from a biography of a jolly British journalist: "It was a life of taverns, of roaring discussions that went on for hour after hour, of articles scribbled on odd sheets of paper wedged on the pub table beside the tankard of beer or the bottle of wine, the printer's boy waiting patiently for the copy, and often the cab standing on the kerb outside, forgotten, the driver pulling the thick rug around his legs to keep warm, and the cab-horse's head drooping into its nosebag; and the gaslamps flaring over the presses, bringing out the issues for the night." Name the poet, author, literary critic, and detective story writer (the Father Brown series) who is the subject of this biography by Dudley Barker?

A. Gilbert K. Chesterton was a remarkable public figure—a journalist, essayist, commentator—a man so articulate and so intellectually astute that he successfully took on George Bernard Shaw, Bertrand Russell, and Clarence Darrow in debate. The man loved beer. When he converted to Catholicism at age 48, at the height of his career, the English Roman Catholic community was ecstatic, and many a tankard of ale was raised to salute the event.

Q. By the 1870s, lager beer had become the dominant brewed beverage among the American drinking public. The name *lager* gives a clue as to why Milwaukee became so prominent in the brewing industry. What advantage did Milwaukee possess?

A. Lager beer refers, in German, to the method whereby the beer was "lagered," or stored for several months in a cool, secure place. The ground below Milwaukee was ideal for a system of specially installed caves wherein the beer could be stored. The caves in many locales became warm during the summer months, and in the age prior to refrigeration, ice had to be used to keep them cool. Providing ice in many areas was a major and expensive problem. Milwaukee, however, had abundant sources of winter lake ice that could be stored for summer use. The ice crop went to saloons, hotels, restaurants, and especially brewers. The Philip Best Brewing Company, with its Mammoth Cave for lagering beer, used 60,000 tons of ice in 1880.

Q. Ask folks for the name of a black entertainer who is also Jewish, and most will come up with the name Sammy Davis, Jr. However, there is another one, not quite so famous to be sure, but well known to jazz fans, especially those who fancy Harlem "stride" piano. Here he describes some of the benefits of his first steady job at Bill Buss's Saloon in Newark, New Jersey: "Buss would give all the employees three checks when they came to work, good for three beers and a shot of whiskey. You started off with a 'Y-Z' made up of a shot of bar booze and a short beer chaser. After that, you still had two regular beers coming with your checks." Who was this 14-year-old piano prodigy, eventually to be a Hebrew cantor of deep faith?

A. The autobiography is called *Music on My Mind,* and the musician author is one of the four greats of Harlem stride piano (the other three being Fats Waller, Jelly Roll Morton, and Jimmy the Brute Johnson). Willie the Lion Smith became interested in Judaism when he was a small boy, helping his mother deliver the washing and ironing she took in for an income. While delivering to one Jewish family, he overheard the children being taught Hebrew. The family let the Lion sit in. When he was 13, he had his bar mitzvah in a Newark synagogue and he remained Jewish all his life. For a time, he served as a cantor in a Harlem synagogue. Duke Ellington says in the foreword to the Lion's book: "The Lion has been the greatest influence on most of the great piano players. . . . I swam in it. . . . Even the great Art Tatum, as great as he was—and I know he was the greatest—showed strong patterns of Willie Smithisms after being exposed to The Lion."

Q. All beer drinkers are familiar with the term "premium beer" and some have even heard about "super-premium beers." What, exactly, do the terms mean?

A. The most consistent significance of the terms has to do with price: super-premium beers (e.g., Löwenbräu, Michelob, Henry Weinhard, Anchor Steam, Augsberger) tend to cost more than premium beers (e.g., Miller, Bud, Schlitz, Pabst, Stroh's, Coors, Tuborg), which tend to cost more than "popular" brands (e.g., Schlitz, Old Milwaukee, Blatz). The higher-priced labels have a tendency to score higher in blind tastings, but not consistently so; and sometimes some of the most expensive will be regarded as frankly lousy. It used to be (in the 1940s and 1950s) that the term *premium* had some significance. It referred to a product that was brewed elsewhere but, because of aggressive advertising or other factors, was sold at some distance from where it was made. As a consequence, a shipping charge or premium was tacked on, making it more expensive than the local product. Anyway, what is most important is your own judgment in the matter; don't let the classifications or the ratings interfere with your own enjoyment.

Q. If you are a Piel's beer fan and if you are old enough, you may remember a series of TV ads in which the then very popular comedy team of Bob and Ray became spokesmen for the Piel brothers, soft-spoken Harry and loud, overblown Bert. The commercials were not only long-lived, everyone loved them. As it turned out, Bert and Harry made a lot of people talk about Piel's, but beer sales didn't increase at all. The Bert and Harry episode, according to author Lincoln Diamant, became a famous object lesson in advertising circles: entertaining commercials don't necessarily sell the product. You can still buy Piel's beer, of course, but the brothers no longer own it. Who does?

A. The Piel's beer saga is another object lesson in addition to the advertising one. It's almost impossible to figure out who brews what beer these days. So many of the brewers are huge enterprises with a dozen or more labels, and they seem to trade labels among one another like kids with batches of baseball cards. Piel's was absorbed by the Schaefer Brewing Company in the late 1970s. Schaefer was then sucked up by Stroh's, a family-owned brewing company based in Detroit, whose roster of other brands includes Signature Super Premium, Goebel, Old Milwaukee, and Erlanger. When Stroh's took over Schlitz, it went from the seventh-largest to the third-largest brewer in the United States.

Q. Most people could live happily all their lives without knowing about 3.2 beer, but it is a fact of life for people in some states. Colorado, Kansas, Ohio, and South Dakota, for instance, allow 18-year-olds to drink alcoholic beverages, so long as it is 3.2 beer. That accounts for a sizable chunk of the Midwest. Now then, where did the term *3.2 beer* originate?

A. The Eighteenth Amendment forbade all intoxicating liquors. It was the Volstead Act that defined what this meant: any beverage containing more than 0.5 percent alcohol. By Franklin Delano Roosevelt's election, the folly of national Prohibition was apparent to the vast majority of Americans, and FDR in fact campaigned with a Repeal-of-Prohibition plank. However, while the ponderous machinery to repeal a constitutional amendment got into gear, it was possible for Congress to redefine the term *intoxicating liquors* from the highly restrictive standards of the Volstead Act (i.e., more than 0.5 percent alcohol). Expert testimony before Congress emphasized that beer of 3.2 percent alcohol content would be much more palatable than the pre-Prohibition Food Control Bill standard of 2.75 percent, the reason being that highly aromatic and flavorful hop oils are soluble in alcohol and not in water. The slight increase in alcohol content therefore creates a substantial improvement in taste. The passage of the Cullen Beer Bill therefore allowed for the production and sale of 3.2 beer (in states not having their own state prohibition laws), effective April 7, 1933.

Q. If you are or ever have been a churchgoer, you may remember a particular sermon as having especially touched your soul. Christmas, more than any other time, seems to bring out the poetry in the minister, as the following excerpt demonstrates: "They welcomed Him with gifts, too. Not with the sacraments, which were yet to be instituted, but with gifts. I use the word in its symbolic sense. And while not as the lantern-jawed Calvinist, that tried to eradicate from this England of ours the very memory of the feast, that generation of gloom, as the great Chesterton called them. Himself, Chesterton, a great man in all senses of the word, a fat man, jolly in God, as sound a judge of beers as he was of theology." The sermon goes on like that, at some length, but the 600 or so prisoners attending the chapel services apparently liked the service well enough. Who was the Irish literary prisoner who recorded the sermon?

A.   Brendan Behan was 16 years old at the time, and a prisoner in His Majesty's Prison in Liverpool. That's what comes of being caught with gelignite and various other explosive paraphernalia. Members of the IRA weren't very popular in the prisons—neither with the guards nor with the other prisoners—but Behan was such a personable and self-sufficient lad that he got along just fine. On food and drink, he had this to say: "As regards drink, I can only say that in Dublin, during the depression when I was growing up, drunkenness was not regarded as a social disgrace. To get enough to eat was regarded as an achievement. To get drunk was a victory."

Q.   There was a lovely little short story called "Past One at Rooney's" that captured a bit of American morals in transition at the turn of the century. "Rooney's is more than respectable by daylight; stout ladies with children and mittens and bundles and unpedigreed dogs drop up of afternoons for steins and a chat." But at night, Rooney's was a very different place, because Rooney was twenty years ahead of his time: after twilight, Rooney allowed women to smoke! "A girl alone entered Rooney's, glanced around with leisurely swiftness, and sat opposite McManus at his table. Her eyes rested upon him for two seconds in the look with which woman reconnoiters all men whom she for the first time confronts. In that space of time, she will decide on one of two things—either to scream for the police, or that she may marry him later on. . . . After she had ordered a small beer from the immediate waiter, she took from her bag a box of cigarettes and lighted one with slightly exaggerated manner. Then she looked again into the eyes of Cork McManus and smiled. Instantly, the doom of each was sealed." Who is the famous short story writer at work here?

A.   William S. Porter could pack more character and more story into a few pages than anyone before or since. He's more familiar to most folks under his pen name of O. Henry. There's a lot of beer in many of his stories—and wine and whiskey and rum as well—and he often used taverns and bars and saloons as the settings for his tales, many of which were distinguished by a surprise twist for an ending (as certainly was true in "Past One at Rooney's"). He was one of the highest paid and most prolific writers of his day when he died in New York in 1910 of tuberculosis.

Q.   Altogether, there are thirteen countries in South America, half a dozen in Central America, and three more in North America. In total, they account for a lot of beer production and a lot of beer consumption. Now, which one of them has the most puritanical drinking laws?

A.   It may come as a surprise to those Americans who fancy the robust flavors of Canadian brews to learn that the quality of these beverages is *not* a function of a permissive government attitude. While prohibition had a rather haphazard application in Canada, its effects on Canadian social habits has been persistent. In most places, buying a beer on Sunday is difficult, if not impossible. Until the 1950s, Canadians needed annual permits before they could buy drinks at all. Canada has many "dry" areas (e.g., Saskatchewan) and in general it is impossible to buy packaged goods except from rigidly controlled government stores.

DAY 10 DIET

It's funny how one's mood changes. I'm feeling a lot more optimistic about Wednesdays than I did last week at this time. The world seems a gentler, more felicitous place. In this nearly happy frame of mind, I think of Wednesdays as the kind of day in which the first-ever father-and-son team shot a hole in one on the same hole in the same game. That would be Charles H. Calhoun, Sr. and Jr., at the third hole, Washington Golf Club, Washington, Georgia, on August 24, 1932.

Approach this diet day with the confidence that it's going to be a winning dawn-to-dusk for you and all the people you care about.

BREAKFAST:

If you are a morning paper reader, you may have noticed that Wednesdays are often big days for grocery advertisements, special food sections with lots of recipes, and the like. Don't fear. You can now allow yourself to start imagining what life will be like after the diet is over. Just remember to begin the day with 12 ounces of water, your multivitamin, and a thiamine tablet.

The Menu   **Puffed Rice (1 cup), seasoned with
cinnamon and artificial
sweetener
Skim milk (¼ cup)
Vegetable Juice (6 ounces)
Coffee or Tea, as you like**

MIDMORNING:

Coffee break is coffee break. It's not a party, but then what did you expect? If you are a tea drinker, try a new tea bag for a change.

LUNCH:

Among folks who like pilsener beer, the brew from Czechoslovakia is simply unbeatable. Pilsner Urquell calls itself "the oldest beer in the world," dating from 1292; and in its honor we will borrow from Czech cuisine for our lunch today. Don't forget to have a large glass of water before sitting down to dine.

**The Menu   Chef's Choice Lunch: Czech-style
Cabbage**

1 pound red cabbage
¼ cup unsweetened applesauce
2 tablespoons lemon juice
1 teaspoon sugar
1 teaspoon all-purpose flour
½ teaspoon salt
1 tablespoon caraway seeds
1 tablespoon vinegar

Wash and shred the cabbage into fine strips. Combine with the other ingredients and stir well. Cook over low heat, stirring from time to time until tender (about 20–30 minutes). Serve and enjoy.

The Menu   Restaurant Lunch: Veggies, Bohemian-style

If you live in an area where there are a lot of Eastern Europeans, you should not have much difficulty finding a restaurant that serves Czech food. Unfortunately, these are not exactly your basic diet-food establishments; and it is entirely possible that there is nothing on the menu that you can get for under 200 calories. Your best bets will be soups—if not too meaty or starchy—or veggies, particularly cabbage dishes, if not prepared with heavy doses of animal fats and sour cream dressings. Careful, friend.

The Menu   Brown Bag Lunch: Sweet and Sour Cabbage

There are a number of brands of sweet-and-sour-style cabbage on the market. This is typical Czech fare, quite tasty and filling as well. Typical examples include Greenwood's (in a can) and Lord Mott's (in a jar). You can have a cup and a half of either. Simply put the contents in a microwave-safe container and press the appropriate button.

MIDAFTERNOON:

Do your usual fluids number with some ice water, diet soft drink, club soda, or coffee or tea. Sneak a peek at the Diversion Quiz if your thoughts turn to food.

SUPPER:

The Australians are, of course, great beer drinkers, and many Americans like the robust Australian brews. Great beer drinkers and great beer producers! In their honor, it seems only fair to have a meal that samples their cuisine. This is not as easy as it sounds. Witness this excerpt from John Gunther's *Inside Australia*:

> Until the food-conscious immigrants came, Australian food was confined, pretty much everyone agrees, to steak and eggs. Cyril Pearl offers a tongue-in-cheek recipe: "Take a piece of old bullock, cut as thin as possible, throw into a frying-pan with a spoonful of sump-oil (winter grade is preferable) and burn to the ground. Fry an egg in same oil. When both are cold, toss on to a soapy plate and cover with tomato sauce."

In order to eat tastily in an Australian fashion, therefore, we need to turn to one of Australia's many immigrant groups. The big continent down under has not always provided a receptive doorway to Asian peoples, but the Chinese style of cooking provides one of its finest dinners. Be sure to have your regulation 12 ounces of water before dinner.

The Menu   Chef's Choice Dinner: Stir-fry Chicken

The Chinese stir-fry method of cooking is simple and quick, and it's even kind of fun. It is also great for making a small amount of meat stretch a long way, and therefore easy on your pocketbook as well as good for your diet. Try this dish with an Australian brew, or even one of the growing number of brands available from China.

2 tablespoons soy sauce
5 garlic cloves, minced
2–3 fresh ginger slices (if you can get the ginger)
1 teaspoon cornstarch
¼ pound chicken breast, skinless, sliced in
   strips (pencil thickness)
½ cup frozen green peas
¼ sweet red pepper, cut in narrow strips
1 teaspoon vegetable oil
¼ pound fresh mushrooms, cleaned and sliced
2 green onions, including the green part, cut
   into 1" segments
1 ounce water chestnuts, sliced thinly
   Salt and pepper to taste

Combine the soy sauce, garlic, ginger, and cornstarch into a smooth, thick solution. Add the sliced chicken breast, mix thoroughly, and allow to set for 1–2 hours (a small plastic bag is good for this). Meanwhile, put the green peas and red peppers into a small amount of boiling, salted water for 2–4 minutes (or until barely tender); then remove, saving the water separately. When the chicken has marinated for an hour or two, put the oil in a nonstick pan, place on medium heat and sauté the mushrooms and chicken, stirring rapidly, until browned (about 3–5 minutes). Then add several tablespoons of the water you used to cook the veggies, stirring all the while, and add the peas, peppers, onions, and water chestnuts. Season to taste. When the whole mixture is warmed throughout, it is ready. Get out the chopsticks and attack! Delicious!

The Menu   Restaurant Dinner: Stir-fry

If your town doesn't have an Australian restaurant handy (and it's not bloody likely outside of Australia itself), then take yourself out to your local Chinese place and count your blessings. Such establishments are great for dieters, so long as you limit yourself to one entree, avoiding the pork and the rice. Your best bet is a stir-fry of chicken or shrimp with veggies, e.g., snowpeas, mushrooms, beans, and the like. No oyster sauce, friend, and stay away from restaurants that use so much cornstarch that the ingredients look pasted together.

The Menu   Brown Bag Dinner: Chinese Frozen Dinner

If you are brown bagging it today, go to a little extra effort to spruce up the place where you will be eating. Bring a fancy napkin and your favorite beer glass. Buy a brew that is a little special. For the food, let me recommend one of Chun King's 11-ounce chow mein dinners—the beef or the chicken or the shrimp. They also produce an egg foo yung platter (also 11 ounces), which falls within our range. If none of these strike your fancy, try one of the frozen dinners recommended on Day 4. Eat with chopsticks, if you can!

EVENING:

If you haven't already polished off your quota of brews for the day, now is the time to do so. Have a glass of water before each beer, find an easy chair, and show off with the Diversion Quiz.

DAY **10** DIVERSIONS

Q. Americans are often intrigued and amused by the way Australians talk. One of the reasons for the popularity of the song "Waltzing Matilda" in the United States is that so many of the words seem absolutely improbable. I remember being taken aback when an Australian woman started talking about "drinking piss and sucking fags." What was she implying?

A. She was referring to a popular Australian pastime, drinking beer and smoking cigarettes. John Gunther gives us some insight into more Australian slang in *Inside Australia*: "Barmaids are collectively a precious Australian tradition—cheery women who josh the customers as they fill a glass, let the head subside, top it off with more beer, and serve it. 'Seventeen cents, thank you, love.' Their expression for a repeat is 'something similar,' on the indisputable grounds that you can't have the 'same' drink that you just drank. Treating in Australianese is 'shouting'—'I'll shout you a beer'—the best guess about the origin of the expression is that rich, expansive, gold miners used to shout for everyone in the neighborhood to come to the pub and have a beer."

Q. Most people think they know what fermentation is: a process that results in beer. But as Beatrice Hunter points out in *Fermented Foods and Beverages*, lots of other things are products of fermentation, too: sauerkraut, champagne, bread, vinegar, pickles, tofu, and lots more. What, exactly, is fermentation?

A. Fermentation refers to a process whereby yeasts—which are single-celled living organisms—break down sugars to produce energy and nutrients conducive to their own growth and reproduction. Alcohol production is produced when the fermentation is largely anaerobic, i.e., when no oxygen is present. Aerobic fermentation (i.e., with lots of oxygen, as in bread making) involves a more complete form of chemical processing in which whatever alcohol is produced is further broken down to oxygen and water.

Q. Here's a tough one. Even if you can't guess it exactly, see how close you can come. What kind of beer are we talking about and where does the story take place in this tale called "Puborama," by Don MacKay:

> A fisherman from the city was waylaid by an aggressive-looking bushman who carried a bottle in one hand and a shotgun in the other. "Here, sport," said the bushman, "have a drink on me!" The angler protested that he didn't drink. Leveling his gun at him, the owner of the bottle ordered, "Drink!" The man from the city drank, then shuddered, shook, shivered and coughed mightily. "Well," he spluttered, "that's horrible stuff!"
>
> "Ain't it?" agreed the bushman. "Now you hold the gun on me while I take a gulp!"

A. This particular story is taken from *A Book of New Zealand* and stems from the King Country in New Zealand—though in truth similar tales derive from other nations as well. The beverage was Matai beer, the recipe for which depended upon adding three or four cupfuls of yellow pine sap to a gallon of ordinary brew. "Matai beer . . . may be identified easily. It smells like an ancient bar room the morning after. It tastes like used machine oil, only a very low-grade of machine oil. When a deep swig is absorbed, one has all the sensations of having swallowed a lighted kerosene stove. A sudden violent jolt of it has been known to stop the victim's watch, snap his braces, and crack his glass eye right across—all in the same motion. If it must be drunk, drink it while sitting flat on the floor. Then you don't have so far to fall."

Q. If you had been in Jackson Hole, Wyoming, in the early 1950s, while Donald Hough was doing research for his book *The Cocktail Hour in Jackson Hole,* you would probably have met a colorful fellow named Dews, who lived in the basement of the Silver Dollar Saloon. "There he had a corner space, or apartment, two walls of which were formed by stacks of beer cases reaching almost to the ceiling. . . . He went to his north wall and extracted a hunting knife from between two cases, then turned to me. 'Schlitz, Coors, Rainier, Acme, Pabst, Sheridan, Budweiser—just name it.' " I think my fridge is well stocked, but who can compete with that larder? Now, tell me where you would go to find the breweries that produce Rainier, Acme, and Sheridan?

A. The Rainier Brewing Company in Seattle was bought out just before its hundredth anniversary in 1977 by Heileman. You can still purchase the Rainier brand, however, and I would particularly commend Rainier Ale, a heavy-bodied, well-hopped brew, especially favored by the late San Francisco columnist Charles McCabe, and called by him the Green Death. (He finished off five of the green cans every day.) Acme was a San Francisco firm that was bought out by Rheingold in 1954. There was a Sheridan Brewery in Sheridan, Wyoming, until at least the mid-1950s, and another in Pueblo, Colorado, until at least the early 1970s. Neither is currently operating.

Q. You probably took some chemistry classes some place along the way, so I'm going to test you on a few terms. What do the following have in common: (1) heptylparaben, (2) enocianina, (3) jasmine oil, (4) sodium metabisulfite, (5) proplylene glycol alginate, (6) bromelain, and (7) diastase?

A.   According to a little book called *Chemical Additives in Booze,* all of these chemicals (plus 60 or so others) have been approved by the Bureau of Alcohol, Tobacco and Firearms, as acceptable additives in beer. In order, they are used as: (1) an antimicrobial preservative, (2) an artificial coloring agent, (3) a flavoring additive, (4) an antioxidant, (5) a foam-stabilizing and anti-gushing agent, (6) a clarifier and chillproofer, and (7) an enzyme that helps convert starch to sugar. Most brewers use one or more of these additives, though a few use none at all. If current proposed regulations go into effect as expected in 1984, all such additives will have to be listed on the label.

Q.   If you travel much in the Orient, you will notice that the business communities in many Asian countries—Malaya, the Philippines, Burma—include large numbers of Chinese, far out of proportion to their percentages in the general population. In addition, the Chinese children tend to be aggressive competitors when faced with academic challenges; and Chinese families are known for their strong sense of community. During the colonial era, some Westerners noted these qualities and, correctly or incorrectly, referred to the Chinese as "the Jews of the Orient." With this rather lengthy, apparent digression, can you guess which beverage company the Chinese chose to be sole importers of their Tsingtao beer when they started shipping to this country in 1978?

A.   According to a story in the *New Yorker,* the exclusive U.S. importers of Tsingtao beer have been the Monarch Wine Company of Brooklyn, which also happens to be bottlers of Manischewitz brand kosher sacramental wine. Leo Star, the 81-year-old president of Monarch, flew to China to sign the deal, and the Chinese were pleased and honored that the patriarch flew so far. They also reportedly were pleased that Monarch is a family operation, run not only by Mr. Star but also by his three sons-in-law. Respect for family and for age, combined with Yankee ingenuity and hard work, clinched the deal. In 1981, a million cases of Tsingtao were sold in the United States.

Q. I know a lovely woman who likes beer, but won't drink it because it gives her gas. She was brought up in a time and place where girls aspired to be ladies, and ladies were never troubled by gaseousness. Not all people are so affected, and of those who are, some take advantage of the situation. Who is the famous baseball hero, Baltimore-born, brought up in an orphanage, who—pointing to a silver cup—spoke these enduring lines: "Look at this one, you know what I got it for?! I won first place in a farting contest! Honest. Read the writing on it. Boy, I had to down a lot of beer and limburger to win that one!"

A. Babe Ruth was that kind of fellow: coarse, open, full of life and food and drink and enthusiasm. Robert Creamer describes him beautifully in his book *Babe*. The book also includes this story told by Ty Cobb: "I've seen him at midnight, propped up in bed, order six club sandwiches, a platter of pigs' knuckles, and a pitcher of beer. He'd down all that while sucking a big, black cigar. Next day, if he hit a homer, he'd trot around the bases complaining about gas pains and a bellyache." Creamer says Ruth belched magnificently and could fart at will.

Q. If you look at a map of Brazil, you'll find a lot of rivers feeding into the Amazon. Among the dozens of Portuguese names, one stands out: Rio Roosevelt. Until 1913, it was known as the Castanho, or, in English, the "river of doubt." During that year, Teddy Roosevelt led an expedition of twenty-two men on a mission of zoologic and geographic discovery. The trip lasted five months, far longer than originally intended, and resulted in the death of one man, with Roosevelt becoming seriously ill with malaria, dysentery, and deep abscesses. Just getting into the river's source, in the high plateau of the Matto Grasso, near the Bolivian border, was quite an expedition in itself, requiring 200 oxen, mules, and horses to transport food, equipment, and of course, beer. Any guesses on what brand T.R. chose to take along?

A.   According to *Fortune* magazine, January 1936, Roosevelt took 24 cases of Schlitz with him—which must have required several oxen all by itself. Schlitz was the nation's second-largest brewer around the turn of the century, just behind Pabst and ahead of Anheuser-Busch, all selling in the million-cases-a-year range. Schlitz's popularity was such that it was a favorite of many notables, a fact that it used in advertisements at the end of Prohibition. Among others, the ads mentioned that Admiral George Dewey distributed 3,600 bottles of Schlitz among his sailors after he captured Manila Bay.

Q.   If you visit a fair number of beer emporiums over the course of the year, you undoubtedly have encountered little mats or coasters just large enough to accommodate the bottom of a beer mug. Most of them are decorated with an advertisement for a brand of beer, though some plug a particular saloon. Any guesses how long these little treasures have been decorating saloon tables?

A.   The first wood-pulp-style beer mat or coaster was patented in 1892 by Robert Sputh in Dresden, Germany. Collectors of the genre (or tegestologists, as they call themselves, from the Latin *teges*, meaning a covering or mat), are now common in many countries. An Austrian, Leo Pisker, is credited with having the world's largest collection, with approximately 70,000 mats.

Q.   These days, when we hear the terms *cocktail* and *mixed drink*, we tend to think in terms of distilled beverages with some sort of mixer or occasionally we think of some wine concoction. However, brewed beverages have long been used in mixed drinks, too. How many of the following can you identify: black velvet, shandy (or shandy gaff), lamb's wool, syllabub, beer flip?

A. The black velvet is composed of chilled, equal parts of stout (usually Guinness) and champagne. The shandy sounds terrible, but actually is a decent hot-weather drink. The original recipe called for equal parts of lemonade and strong beer, but I've seen versions that call for ginger ale and British ale. Lamb's wool is a traditional English Christmas drink, *the* beverage to put in your wassail bowl, and generally includes "nut-brown ale," roasted crab apples, sugar, nutmeg, and ginger. The traditional syllabub called for strong ale, sugar, nutmeg, and milk *directly from the cow's udder*, with the teats milked rapidly to raise a good foam. The beer flip has numerous variations, but one popular recipe asks you to boil a quart of beer, then beat in an egg or three, and add such flavorings as a glass of gin, sugar, cinnamon, and lemon juice.

Q. If you looked at the sales records of the top five beverage companies in the United States, together their annual sales would amount to over $16 billion. Can you identify the companies?

A. Anheuser-Busch is number one, with sales of $4.7 billion (according to *Beverage World,* July 1983), but that is only because Coca-Cola sales are divided up among Coca-Cola Bottling of New York, Mid-Atlantic Coca-Cola, etc. The number-two outfit is Coca-Cola Company (of Atlanta, Georgia), which includes in its beverage sales Minute Maid juices, Taylor California wines, Sterling wines, and Monterey brand wines. The number-three company is, of all things, Phillip Morris, whose beverage empire includes Miller Brewing and Seven-Up. Number four is Seagram's, who, in addition to the obvious booze line, also owns Calvert whiskeys and Paul Masson wines, among others. In the number-five spot is Pepsi Company of

Purchase, New York (which would be higher on the list if it produced all the Pepsi, which it doesn't, since there are numerous other Pepsi bottlers scattered around the country).

Q. When brewers hype their beer, a common claim to individuality and excellence concerns the water from which the beer is brewed. That has certainly been the approach of the Olympic Brewing Company with its artesian springs in Tumwater, Washington; and Hamm's likewise has spent untold millions touting "the Land of Sky Blue Waters." What brewery attributes the fine taste of its beer to the waters of Mt. Lao?

A. For this item, we are indebted to *The China Guidebook,* written by Frederick Kaplan and Arne de Keijzer:

> Qingdao Brewery. Perhaps one of the few positive legacies of Western Colonialism in China is Qingdao's Brewery, established by the Germans at the turn of the century. Some of the old wooden machinery is still in use, although it is being supplanted by glistening new bottling machines recently imported from the Federal Republic of Germany. Instead of the usual "briefing with tea," visitors to the brewery will get a "briefing with beer," served ice-cold in the traditional green bottles. . . .
>
> Although there are favorite brands in China (Wuxing in Beijing, Baiyun in Guangzhou, and the somewhat watery Shanghai brand), Qingdao beer is the most popular for export (it is sold under the old name, Tsingtao, in the U.S.). Its fine flavor is attributable to the water from Mt. Lao (Laoshan), which also produces the best-known mineral water in China.

Q. Think of the company that for a number of years was the third-largest brewing company in the world (currently ranking about sixth place), and you should automatically think of a color intimately connected with its trademark. Name that company.

A. While Pabst began using the words "blue ribbon" in 1895 in connection with its Select brand, the familiar brand name did not actually replace Select until 1897. However, blue ribbons had been tied around the necks of bottles of Select since 1882. As the beer became more popular, huge amounts of silk ribbon were required; over 300,000 yards were tied around necks of Select in 1892 alone.

Q. Brewers are people with passions, just like other ordinary human beings. Sometimes they enjoy celebrating something that seems a bit special to them. Sometimes they get carried away by fads and popular enthusiasms, and sometimes they shrewdly try to profit from the quirks and interests of others. So it is that brewers from time to time put out special commemorative beers. In 1955, a New Zealand brewer produced a series of special brews to commemorate, and to supply, what was then, in those pre-spaceflight days, considered to be man's last great adventure in exploration. Any guesses what that might be?

A. The brand was Bavarian Old Style Lager, but the cans were marked "specially for Operation Deep Freeze," Admiral Richard E. Byrd's epic adventure in the Antarctic. Such novelty and exotic cans drive beer can collectors wild. United Air Lines commissioned a Brew 747 to promote its flights to Hawaii. Continental Can issued a special label in 1975 in honor of its twenty-fifth year in Milwaukee. The Master Brewers Association issued a special can for its thirty-sixth annual convention in San Francisco. The list goes on and on.

Q. When you consider the 20 million barrels of beer produced annually by Anheuser-Busch, the small, so-called boutique breweries scattered across the country don't amount to very much. Still, they add a special regionalized spice to a beer drinker's consumption, and most of us enjoy a taste of something new and unique, brewed by some dedicated artist scratching out a living in a small workshop someplace. Many of them are marginal operations when you look at their balance sheets, operational only so long as the owner is willing to get by on a subsistence basis. How many brewers can you name who produce less than 10,000 barrels a year?

A. The answer to this question may be outdated before it reaches print, because some companies are born and die so rapidly. In the last year, New Albion and DeBakker (both in California) have faded out of existence, and I have heard rumors of a couple of others in California that are due to start up. At this writing, Anchor Steam Brewing Company in San Francisco is no longer a micro-brewer, now producing over 28,000 barrels. True micro-brewers include Sierra Nevada (Chico, California—2,000 barrels); River City (Sacramento, California—3,000 barrels); Thousand Oaks (Berkeley, California—about 500 barrels); New Amsterdam (Utica, New York—2,500 barrels); Real Ale (Ann Arbor, Michigan—600 barrels); Red Hook Brewery (Seattle, Washington—3,000 barrels); William S. Newman Company (Albany, New York—2,000 barrels); and my favorite local, Buffalo Bill's Brewery (Hayward, California—about 300 barrels). Others, on which I lack production data, include: Grants, in Yakima, Washington; Boulder Brewery, in Colorado; Hale's, in Coleville, Washington; Jones Brewing, in Smithton, Pennsylvania; Hopland, in Hopland, California; and Horse Shoe Bay Brewery (but that's actually across the border in British Columbia).

Q. You know the combination bottle and can opener, rounded at one end and sharp at the other, that punches a triangular hole in the top of beverage cans? I've always called it a church key, and so do my friends. However, finding the origin of the term has been a real challenge. Most of the librarians I consulted had never heard the term (they admitted they weren't beer drinkers), and over two dozen books on word usage, slang, and jargon were no help at all. Any guesses where the term *church key* originates?

A. The expression *church key* has been around for many years, according to *The Dictionary of Word and Phrase Origins*. The term originally referred to a heavy cast-iron bottle opener, used to pry off metal crowns, which had a circular open end that resembled the handle of large, heavy keys used to open massive church doors. The term *church key* springs from this resemblance. "With the coming of cans in the brewing business, the bottle opener gave way to the can opener that makes the triangular marks—but the name church key was simply transferred to the new device."

DAY **11** DIET

Sweet Thursday follows lousy Wednesday, as John Steinbeck once noted, and Maundy Thursday precedes Good Friday. Maundy Thursday, for those of us unschooled in such things, is a day traditionally marked by acts of charity and humility, best exemplified by the British monarch who would summon poor folk—as many as the king or queen was years old—and would wash their feet and gift them with baskets (called "maunds") of food. Maybe this day won't be so terrible after all.

BREAKFAST:

Step number one: get out of bed. Step number two: spend the required amount of time in the bathroom. Drink your full 12 ounces of water and down your multivitamin and thiamine tablets. When you are dressed, proceed to breakfast.

The Menu   **Blackberries (1 cup, fresh or
canned in water)
Coffee or Tea, till you feel full and
reasonably alert**

MIDMORNING:

More coffee or tea, friend. If you are tempted by doughnuts, sweet rolls, and the like, distract yourself with some items from the Diversion Quiz.

LUNCH:

What came first, the chicken or the egg? Well, last night you had chicken, so for lunch we will have eggs. Lovely little items, eggs are. Almost everyone knows how to cook them in some fashion, and they are even reasonably low in calories—the medium size running about 70 calories and the extra-large, about 90. The biggest problem with eggs is that most people have them fried, with lots of butter—and oftentimes with other fattening goodies—so we'll need to keep that in mind as we proceed. Be sure to begin lunch with your 12-ounce glass of water.

The Menu   Chef's Choice Lunch: Western Omelet

There are a wide variety of recipes that fit under the general title of "western omelet." This one needs to be a two-egg omelet to fit within the 200-calories lunch limit. Add or subtract herbs, celery, and green onion to suit your taste.

>   Nonstick cooking spray
> 2   green onions, chopped
> ½   stalk celery, chopped
> ½   tomato, seeded and chopped
> 1   dash hot sauce
>   Salt and pepper to taste
> 2   medium-size eggs
> ½   teaspoon oregano

Spray a frying pan with nonstick spray, and gently sauté the onion, celery, tomato, hot sauce, salt, and pepper, until barely softened and tender. Set aside and keep warm. Then spray the pan again. Beat the eggs thoroughly with the oregano, and heat in the frying pan. When the eggs are cooked, place the vegetable mixture in the center, fold the eggs to encase the veggies, and serve.

The Menu   Restaurant Lunch: Omelet

In a restaurant, you almost inevitably will go over 200 calories, but if you are careful, it will be close enough to be acceptable. Ask for a two-egg omelet instead of the more common three-egg version. Explain that you are on the I-Like-My-Beer Diet, and that, if the chef uses a bare minimum of butter, you can have a beer. A beer-drinking waiter or waitress will almost certainly understand and urge the chef to comply. The safest omelet to have is a plain one, but the veggies put into the standard western omelet are probably okay if not sautéed with butter. Remember to avoid bread and potatoes.

The Menu   Brown Bag Lunch: Hard-boiled Eggs
Veggies

It's not easy to brown bag eggs. There are some frozen egg-and-sausage dinners, but they average double our calorie limit, and an egg foo yung frozen dinner is almost as bad. Your best bet is to hard-boil two eggs (or buy them already cooked at your local deli or sandwich counter), cut them into quarters, sprinkle with salt and pepper, and take your time eating them. Don't gulp each in one bite. In addition, supply yourself with carrot and celery sticks and green onions to munch on. Not the greatest lunch of all time, but satisfactory. Besides, you're almost through with this damn diet!

MIDAFTERNOON:

Take your break this afternoon with the usual beverages. To add a note of interest, try one or more diet drinks you have never tasted before. Approach the experiment objectively. Make a list of all the things you hate about diet drinks.

SUPPER:

It's Happy Hour time! If you managed to skip the beer earlier in the day, now is the time to give yourself a treat. Get a bottle of your favorite brew and allow yourself to relax. Of course, have a full glass of water first. Tonight we'll borrow a stanza from the Reverend Sydney Smith to set the tone for our dinner:

On the table spread the cloth,
Let the knives be sharp and clean,
Pickles get and salad both,
Let them each be fresh and green.
With small beer, good ale, and wine,
O ye gods! how I shall dine!

We'll skip the wine, but you are welcome to a dill pickle, if you wish. However, the main event will be a seafood salad.

The Menu   Chef's Choice Dinner: Seafood Salad

With most vinegar, you need oil to balance the tartne₋₋ when you use it to dress a salad. Not so with rice vinega which is much milder and available in Oriental market ᴜ sometimes the fancy foods section of supermarket· Rɪᴄʀ vinegar is quite mild, and comes either plain or seasoₙed With the plain (used in the recipe here) you need to add a bit of sugar, but the absence of oil makes this a delightful low-calorie meal. If you use seasoned rice vinegar, you can eliminate the sugar, salt, and pepper.

> 1 head Boston or Bibb lettuce, washed and
>   drained
> 1 large cucumber, peeled and sliced
> 1 tomato, sliced
> 4 ounces radishes, sliced (optional)
> ¼ pound cooked crabmeat
> ¼ pound cooked shrimp
> ¼ cup rice vinegar
> 2 teaspoons sugar
> ½ teaspoon salt
> ½ teaspoon pepper (or more, as desired)
>   Sprigs of parsley or coriander

Arrange the lettuce on a plate and distribute the cucumber, tomato, and radishes around the edge. Put the crabmeat and shrimp in the center. Combine the vinegar, sugar, salt, and pepper, and shake well. Pour the mixture over the seafood and vegetables and chill an hour or so before serving. Garnish with parsley or coriander.

The Menu   Restaurant Dinner: Seafood Salad

It's back to a seafood restaurant tonight. Fortunately, most of these have so much in the way of tasty choices that fit within our 400-calorie limit, that this needn't be a burden at all. A good choice would be crab or shrimp Louis, but instead of the rich French or Thousand Island dressing, go for lemon juice. Tell the waiter to take away the bread and butter, and bring lots of lemon wedges instead.

The Menu   Brown Bag Dinner: Seafood Dinner

Instead of trying to brown bag a seafood salad, you get to have the seafood, but without all the green stuff around it. There are lots of choices, so long as you avoid deep-fried items. Stouffer has a number of selections that I can recommend, my preference being their frozen scallops and shrimp mariner (10¼ ounces), but either their lobster Newburg or shrimp Newburg (each 6½ ounces) falls within our calorie limit, too.

EVENING:

If you haven't had your full quota of beer today, now is the time to drink up. Let your seafood dinner put you in the mood to dream of a vacation by the sea. If the dream disappears before your beer does, finish up the Diversion Quiz for the day.

DAY 11 DIVERSIONS

Q. You probably didn't get a chance to leaf through it in your local bookstore, but one of the most highly touted publishing "events" of recent years was the publication of *The Plan of St. Gall*. The three-volume work, published by the University of California Press (price $450), details the design of a self-contained monastic community. The plans themselves date from A.D. 820, though the Swiss Benedictine monastery had been established some 200 years earlier by the Irish monk Gallus. Now then, if you are a true beer nut, what you'll look for in this marvelous document, this relic of a profoundly civilized intelligence, is some sign that the good monks drank beer. What evidence would you seek, to satisfy yourself?

A. Of course the good monks drank beer. By the year 820 almost all monasteries produced beer. There is evidence that each friar received a ration of a gallon a day. The monks apparently brewed a potent beer for themselves and honored guests, and a weaker concoction for less distinguished visitors. The plans themselves show a brewer's granary and no less than *three* brewing areas. There is the Monks' Bake and Brew House, the Kitchen Bake and Brew House for Distinguished Guests, and the Kitchen Bake and Brew House for Paupers and Pilgrims.

Q. If you go to the fourth-largest zoo in the United States, you'll find some sociable orangutans who will beg to have beer dribbled into their mouths from the bridge over their island. You may think it is demeaning for George and Skinny to behave in such a fashion, but consider the reward: not only do they get the beer, but the zoo owners are mightily pleased, since they happen to be brewers themselves. What Florida brewer built a now world-famous zoo in Tampa in 1959, to pacify the locals for erecting a brewery so near the state university?

A. When Auggie Busch built Busch Gardens, he was able to stock it with exotic birds from the Busch family collection. This fledgling effort was so successful that Anheuser-Busch set up a whole entertainment division and converted the bird garden into a major 300-acre amusement park and zoo. The place showcases over 3,000 mammals, bird and reptiles, featuring many exotic species, and a very successful reproduction program. If you pay the park admission, you get to quaff free beer in the beer garden that still occupies one corner of the park.

Q. The following sequence is from a novel called *The Trumpet Major*, one of the lesser works of an author much read in English literature classes. He's talking about Casterbridge "strong beer": "It was of the most beautiful colour that the eye of an artist in beer could desire; full in body, yet brisk as a volcano; piquant, yet without twang; luminous as an autumn sunset; free from streakiness of taste; but, finally rather heady. The masses worshipped it, the minor gentry loved it more than wine, and by the most illustrious country families it was not despised." Can you name this author?

A. Thomas Hardy is better known as the author of *The Return of the Native, Jude the Obscure,* and *Tess of the D'Urbervilles.* It was said of him: "The man could not look out at a window without seeing something that had never been seen before." If you go to England and visit Dorchester (the model for Casterbridge), you may be able to taste some Thomas Hardy's Ale, brewed irregularly by the Eldridge Pope Brewery and distributed in 6.34-ounce "nip" bottles, each bottle with its own serial number prominent on the label. It's a unique brew, supposedly one that will continue to improve in the bottle for twenty-five years.

Q. The alcohol concentration of beer is regulated by state law in many areas. In order to have a malt beverage that is somewhat more zingy than the standard 3.5 percent alcohol concentration present in most beers, some brewing companies market stronger beers under a term the government will accept, "malt liquor," the most widely known of which is Country Club. What was the first malt liquor?

A. In the early 1940s, the Gluek Brothers Brewing Company created a light-colored brew of 7.2 percent alcohol. The Bureau of Alcohol, Tobacco and Firearms refused to let the company call its brew Gluek's Stout, saying that stout had to be dark in color. In 1943, the name was changed to Gluek's Stout to appease the government, but it was officially our first malt liquor. It was marketed in green bottles and cans, and was locally referred to as the "green death." Gluek Brewing went out of business in 1964, and the brand name was sold first to G. Heileman and then to the Cold Stream Brewing Company, but faded into disuse by 1976.

Q. Many taverns have been important as places in which history took place. Fraunces Tavern in New York City, a place you can still visit today, was the setting for George Washington's farewell to his officers after the Revolutionary War. Cromwell first plotted to overthrow the king of England at the Bear in Cambridge. The list could become quite long. However, not many taverns have been so notable that their names have become a part of everyday language. Can you think of an expression, which implies that a story is made up or just a bit of nonsense, that is derived from the names of two English inns or taverns?

A. "Just another cock and bull story" actually refers to two pubs at Stony Stratford, north of London. In the mid-eighteenth century, according to John Watney, "the innkeepers of these two inns happened to be devoted rumour mongers. As there was almost continuous war with France at the time, they used to spell out elaborate tales of disaster in the field. Alarmed, travelers would arrive in London with these tales. At first they were believed, but it was soon discovered that anybody who had stopped at either the Cock or the Bull at Stony Stratford tended to be primed with misleading and alarming information. 'Just another Cock-and-Bull story,' people would say as they listened to the latest and most unlikely tale brought in by the travelers."

Q. Do you remember a movie called *The Deer Hunter*? It was a Vietnam era epic starring Meryl Streep, Robert DeNiro, and other fine folk. Talk about a long movie! Anyhow, for some people in the audience, the real star of the show was the beer featured in the tavern, located in a western Pennsylvania steel town, where the principals seemed to spend most of their time. Can you name that brand of beer?

A. The beer was Rolling Rock Premium, a distinctive brew put out by the small, independent Latrobe Brewery of Latrobe, Pennsylvania. It's quite popular on the East Coast, in the mid-Atlantic states, and has been known to show up as far away as California. It has sometimes been called "the Coors of the East," not because it tastes the same, but rather because it inspires the same kind of cult loyalty.

Q. If you want to get a university degree in wine making, the place to go in the English-speaking world is the University of California at Davis. Where would you find a university program in brewing?

A.   There are no degree programs in brewing per se in the United States, but UC–Davis does offer a B.S. degree that provides for specialization in fermentation science. There are, however, a couple of technical school programs. The Siebel Institute of Technology in Chicago has a 12-week program in brewing technology (intended primarily for brewing production personnel), and the United States Brewing Academy in Mount Vernon, New York, has a shorter, intensive program for brewing industry people. If it's a university program you want, look to Heriot-Watt University in Edinburgh, Scotland, which offers a B.S. degree in brewing.

Q.   Nowadays, with franchise food places covering the country the way corn silos used to, one can scarcely find a suburban community that doesn't have at least one "beer and beef" or "steak and suds" place. Most of us forget, however, that one popular cut of meat has its origin in, and is named after, a popular establishment for the selling of malt beverages. Can you name it?

A.   For the following, we must thank Flexner's *I Hear America Talking*: "Early Americans drank their beer at home, but the men also drank it at inns, taverns, bars, alehouses, porterhouses, beer cellars (1732, from German *bierkeller*), and beerhouses, which around the 1830s were sometimes simply called houses or homes. . . . Porter was popular in early America and alehouses were sometimes called porterhouses (about 1814, Martin Harrison, the proprietor of a New York City porterhouse, popularized the porterhouse steak)."

Q.   "Barrelhouse," as a descriptive term, refers to a style of piano playing popularized by black American blues musicians in the early twentieth century. The term implies a certain down-and-dirty style, with a heavy left hand, "stomping" out the music. Tunes that come to mind include "Barrelhouse Boogie" (Albert Ammons and Pete Johnson), "Barrelhouse

Blues" (Ma Rainey), "Barrelhouse Stomp" (Bud Freeman), and "Barrelhouse Bessie from Basin Street" (Jule Styne). Now, music lovers, as a place in its own right, what was a barrelhouse?

A. If you guessed it was simply a warehouse for storing barrels, you guessed wrong. Flexner gives us the answer, as he tells us about the growing popularity of beer during and after the Civil War: "Americans were soon talking about the beer jerkers (1863) or beer slingers (1875) who worked at the flourishing beer mills (1879), beerhalls (1882, German *bierhalle*), and the barreled beer dives called barrel houses (1882, soon the term came to mean a saloon where women were available, then a whore-house, and finally a style of jazz played there)."

Q. For a long time, Coors beer was available only in the West, and it became something of a cult phenomenon. It was available on the East Coast only when some dealer bootlegged in a truckload, or when a friend or neighbor traveling out west brought back a case or two in the trunk of the car. In 1975, Henry Kissinger got a lot of attention when he stashed forty cases of Coors in a government cargo plane to bring back to Washington, D.C. Presidents Eisenhower and Ford both used *Air Force One* to transport their Coors. For a while, the company even filed suit to prevent the distribution of its beer in the East. The company was the largest brewery in the world, and there was plenty of beer available. What was the problem? Why did the company resist greater distribution?

A. Coors is the only major brewery that does not pasteurize its beer. The problem has been one of freshness and taste. Coors did not want to sell its beer unless it could be confident of an efficient distribution setup. The company requires all distributors to keep the beer chilled in transport and in warehouses, and retailers are supposed to do the same (but, in my experience, few do). Coors is now available in the West, much of the Midwest and South and the District of Columbia. Much of the Coors mystique has been tarnished by a bitter boycott and strike that started in 1977 over Coors labor practices; and the strongly conservative politics of the company's president, Joseph Coors, has also aroused a lot of indignation. Paul Newman is said to have switched brands on that account, from Coors to Bud.

Q. Most of us don't think much about the words we use or the miscellaneous items that fill our houses. Think for a moment about the ordinary tumbler, the kitchen glass that we are likely to use to drink a run-of-the-mill beer. How do you suppose the tumbler got its name?

A. The original tumblers had rounded bottoms, and date back to early Anglo-Saxon times. The design was such that the glasses could be filled only when they were held and, once filled, could not be set down until emptied—whereupon they tumbled over. Now, in more sedate times, the name has remained; but the rounded bottom has gone the way of the Visigoths.

Q. If you frequent saloons that pride themselves on their fake-English decor, you probably have seen those peculiar drinking vessels known as "ale-yards" or as a "long glass." Many novices have tried to drink from them, but have found it no easy task. Why is it so hard?

A. For the answer, we turn to John Bickerdyke and his admirable classic, *The Curiosities of Ale and Beer*: "The ale-yard is described as a trumpet-shaped glass vessel, exactly a yard in length, the narrow end being closed and expanded into a large ball. Its internal capacity is little more than a pint, and when filled with ale, many a thirsty tyro has been challenged to empty it without taking away his mouth. This is no easy task. So long as the tube contains fluid, it flows out smoothly, but when air reaches the bulb, it displaces the liquor with a splash, startling the toper, and compelling him involuntarily to withdraw his mouth by the rush of the cold liquid over his face and dress."

Q. Over the course of your lifetime, you've probably tasted a wide variety of alcoholic beverages. You know they were alcoholic beverages because it says so right on the label. Whiskey lists the alcohol concentration in "proof." Wine lists the alcohol in percent, usually by volume. How is the information listed on your familiar beer can or beer bottle label?

A. Most people are surprised by this. According to my most recent *Master Brewers Association Blue Book*, the vast majority of beer containers show no statement about alcohol content and, in fact, are prohibited from doing so by state law. The principal exceptions are in those states that allow younger drinkers to consume 3.2 beer; these containers must state "not more than 3.2% alcohol by weight" or something similar. Certain states require that the alcohol concentration be on the label if it exceeds a certain amount (e.g., Arkansas 5 percent, Montana 7 percent, Oklahoma 3.2 percent, Oregon 4 percent). Most other states prohibit such information in all or under most circumstances. Exactly why this is so is not clear to the average beer drinker.

Q. A few years ago, Suds Kroge and Dregs Donnigan visited all 132 bars in their hometown and published *A Beer Drinker's Guide* to all such establishments in their city. The best bars were given a Five-Beer rating. The city in question was known up till the mid-1970s as the Pretzel Capital of the World, and has the additional distinction of being the model for the town of Brewer, familiar to folks who like to read novels by John Updike. Can you name it?

A. The full name for Suds and Dregs' book is *A Beer Drinker's Guide to the Bars of Reading*. Suds and Dregs are high school teachers in Reading, Pennsylvania, and therefore decided not to publish the book under their real names, instead choosing these apt "noms de bière." According to an article in the *New Yorker*, Suds and Dregs had such success with their first publishing venture that they expanded their efforts to include the entire county, visiting 238 bars in order to write *A Beer Drinker's Guide to the Berks.*

Q. It used to be that the number-one beer import into the United States was Löwenbräu, but in 1975 Miller started brewing it in this country, at a considerable reduction in price (and, some would say, in taste quality as well). Tuborg also used to be a fancy Danish import until Carling began brewing it at two locations in the States. Shipping beer from Europe to America, according to *Fortune* magazine, "smacks of economic madness. The costs are staggering. Hundreds of tons of glass, mountains of cardboard, and huge transport fees are required to package and dispatch across thousands of miles of ocean an amber fluid that is itself 90% water." Can you name America's favorite imports?

A. Heineken, from Holland, is far and away America's favorite import, accounting for 40 percent of the import market, selling over 2.5 billion cases a year. In fact, Heineken is, by volume, the largest single item shipped from Europe to the North American shores. Canada has second and fourth places locked up with, respectively, Molson's and Moosehead. The leading German beer in this country is Beck's, in third place with a mere sixth of the volume boasted by Heineken.

DAY **12** DIET

My friend, we have arrived. This is it; the last day of the diet—meaning, of course, that tomorrow we can get back to serious eating again. Fridays are wonderful days for arrivals and for new beginnings. It was on this day of the week (March 10, 1876) that Alexander Graham Bell made the world's first telephone call in what was a glorified intercom message to his assistant: "Mr. Watson, come here, I want you," he said. It was on a Friday that the first radio play-by-play of a baseball game was broadcast. On August 5, 1921, Station KDKA in Pittsburgh kept the world abreast of the excitement while the Pittsburgh Corsairs beat out Philadelphia 8–5. And it was on a Friday, too, that Jackie Robinson became the first black to play major league ball, holding down first base for the Brooklyn Dodgers in an exhibition game against the New York Yankees.

While the real eating begins tomorrow, I think you'll be quite pleased with the food today as well. We have something quite special ahead.

BREAKFAST:

Let's see a gleam in your eye this morning. All the grim realities of dieting days are now almost a thing of the past. You have gotten through eleven of these suckers; this last one will be simplicity itself. Remember to start your day with 12 ounces of water, your multivitamin, and the thiamine tablet.

The Menu   **½ Cantaloupe**
Vegetable Juice (6 ounces)
Coffee or Tea, to your heart's
content

MIDMORNING:

Do your usual number with coffee or tea. A smug grin is the appropriate expression to wear in public. When people ask you why you are looking so pleased with yourself (as, of course, they will), tell them you have triumphed through to the final day of the I-Like-My-Beer Diet.

LUNCH:

We'll have a light lunch today to prepare our palates for a particularly nice meal tonight. Onion soup is always a treat, and makes a particularly pleasing light lunch. Take the obligatory glass of water first.

The Menu   Chef's Choice Lunch: Onion Soup

This is an Americanized low-calorie version of the more famous French classic.

    1 teaspoon butter
    1 medium-size onion, sliced thinly and
        separated into rings
    1 clove garlic, minced
    1 tablespoon bread crumbs
    1 pint beef broth (canned, diluted from
        concentrate, or from powder)
    1 tablespoon Parmesan cheese
      Pepper to taste

Use a nonstick pan. Melt the butter and gently sauté the onion rings and garlic. When the onion is soft and nearly translucent, stir in the bread crumbs. Then add the broth and heat to boiling. Serve in a bowl and sprinkle the cheese on top. Bon appétit!

The Menu   Restaurant Dinner: Hot Soup

You have to use your judgment here. Onion soup is a possibility in a restaurant, but their version is likely to be substantially more calorific than the one described above: more butter, lots of bread in the soup, and piles of cheese. You can blow your whole day's allotment of calories on a small bowl of soup. If you are comfortable asking the waiter to leave out the bread and cheese, go ahead and order the soup, and sprinkle one tablespoon of Parmesan cheese on it when it arrives at the table. That should come fairly close to our 200-calorie limit. Otherwise, order a vegetable soup or consommé.

The Menu   Brown Bag Lunch: Hot Soup

If you like French onion soup, Crosse and Blackwell has a fine canned version, as does Campbell's. You can have three full cups of either. There are, of course, numerous French onion soup mixes (Lipton's, Wyler's, Knorr, etc.) and if you have the facilities, you can prepare the soup according to package directions and have three full cups of any of them.

MIDAFTERNOON:

This is the last day of diet soda, so drink up with a sense of abandon. Sneak a peak at the last Diversion Quiz.

SUPPER:

I don't know what your favorite brand of beer is, but this is clearly the time to pop one open. For myself, nothing beats the home brew that my neighbor and I cook up intermittently in my basement, so I'm going to have one of those. Of course, the 12-ounce glass of water comes first.

Our dinner tonight will be on the elegant side, but not uncomfortably so. This is good beer-drinker's fare, and we have the appropriate literary selection to prove it. As Alice Houston tells us: "In the good old days on the Hood River in Oregon, sturgeon were sometimes caught weighing more than a thousand pounds. Their well-salted caviar was handed out free in Western bar-rooms to perk up drinker's lagging taste for beer."

That's right, we're starting off with caviar. It's expensive, but after all the money saved by not buying meat these past twelve days, why not? After that, we'll turn to Izaak Walton for inspiration: "Come, hostess, dress it [a trout] presently, and get us what other meat the house will afford, and give us some of your best barley wine, the good liquor that our honest forefathers did use to drink of; the drink which preserved their health, and made them live so long and do so many good deeds."

One can make wine from barley and other grains, but barley is at its best when used for beer, and I'm sure old Izaak would agree. Anyway, we're having trout for dinner.

The Menu   Chef's Choice Dinner: Caviar
Steamed
Trout
Green Beans

I've eaten many trout over the years, and the ones surrounded by the greatest overall happiness have been those
that I've caught myself and pan-fried immediately afterwards
over a campfire by some magical stream. However, if the truth
be told, the following method (shown to me by my favorite
woman) results in a much better tasting dish of fish.

> 1 ounce caviar, either sturgeon or salmon, as
>   preferred
> 6–8 leaves lettuce, Boston or Bibb
> 1 trout, 6–7-ounce size, gutted
> 1–2 slices fresh ginger
> 1 green onion, including top and bulb,
>   cleaned
> 1 cup green beans, fresh
> 2–3 lemon wedges
>   Salt and pepper, as desired

For the appetizer, simply put one-half teaspoon of caviar
on each small lettuce leaf and arrange on a plate. Sturgeon
caviar is small, most often black or golden in color, and can
be very expensive. The salmon eggs are larger, orange-colored,
and every bit as delightful to many people. Small Boston lettuce leaves make a good vehicle for the delicate eggs, because
the lettuce itself is generally soft (so you can enjoy the texture
of the eggs) and mild (so you can enjoy the taste).

To prepare the trout, simply stuff the cavity with the ginger
and the folded-up green onion. Then place the stuffed trout
on a rack a few inches above boiling water, and steam for 8–
10 minutes. It is a remarkably simple dish and absolutely delicious. Serve with parboiled green beans, flavored with lemon
juice, salt and pepper.

The Menu Restaurant Dinner: Caviar Trout (poached or steamed) Green Veggies

Many fancy restaurants will have caviar available, and if you ask for lettuce leaves on which to place each bite, the restaurant will almost certainly comply. Most charge for the caviar by the ounce—and since it's going to cost you an arm and a leg anyway, tell them to stop at one ounce. That's all you can afford calorie-wise, too. (If they serve things like chopped eggs alongside, ignore them.) Also, most good seafood restaurants are willing to prepare any fish in any style you prefer. Assuming they have trout, ask that it be poached or steamed with spices, but served without any rich sauces. A dish of peas or green beans on the side (no butter!) should round out the meal nicely.

The Menu Brown Bag Dinner: Caviar Fish Specialty Dinner

There's good news and bad news. The bad news is that there's no way I know of that you can get trout in any frozen dinner. The good news is that there are some great-tasting substitutes, and they are all low-cal enough to allow you a double dose of caviar. Pick up a 2-ounce jar of sturgeon or salmon caviar and a head of Boston or Bibb lettuce. Set out a nice array for yourself of small dollops of caviar decorating the lettuce leaves; and, taking your time, pop them into your mouth one at a time, luxuriating in this special occasion. When you are ready for your entree, I would suggest any of the following items from the Stouffer Lean Cuisine line: filet of fish divan (12⅜ ounces), fish Florentine (9 ounces), or Oriental scallops (11 ounces).

EVENING:

Tomorrow morning you can get back to your usual routine. Tonight, if you haven't had your full quota of beers for the day, now is the time (of course, by now you will automatically have a glass of water first). After you have finished the Diversion Quiz, get up and count all the beer bottles you have accumulated over these twelve days. You should have a full case—or more, if you have imbibed light beer.

Not a bad way to diet, huh? Tomorrow morning, get on the scale. If you have followed the diet faithfully, you will have a pleasant reward.

Of course, you will gain back every pound you have lost, if you run true to form. The trick is to do so gradually, over the course of months, rather than gluttonously gaining it all back in one day or even one week. When you are ready to diet again, *The I-Like-My-Beer Diet* will be here to help you.

DAY **12** DIVERSIONS

Q. Probably the most famous beer drinker of recent years was President Carter's brother, Billy Carter. He claimed to drink two six-packs a day, and no one disputed him. In his book, *Cousin Beedie and Cousin Hot,* Carter's cousin Hugh said: "Billy always had a little contempt for Jimmy for not being a beer drinker like he was. And Billy said, 'Since he's running for President, he drinks scotch, and I never trusted a scotch drinker.' " Billy got a lot of mileage out of his beer image. Of course, he sold a lot of beer to the press while they sat around and listened to his inside dope (his gas station was one of only two places in Plains, Georgia, where beer could be purchased); and he did pretty well with his Billy Beer. What company brewed Billy Beer?

A. Fame is fleeting, but Billy made the most of it for a while. On October 31, 1977, it was Billy Beer Day in Plains, with music, competitions, free beer, and Miz Lillian, mother of Jimmy and Billy, wearing a yellow Billy Beer T-shirt. Miz Lillian refused to drink the stuff, however—she said it gave her diarrhea. Initially, Billy Beer was brewed by the Falls City Brewing Company of Louisville, Kentucky, but by the following year at least three other brewers got into the act: the Cold Spring Brewing Company of Cold Spring, Minnesota; the West End Brewing Company of Utica, New York; and Pearl Brewing Company of San Antonio, Texas. Although all the beers were marketed in similar cans, the recipes were apparently different. Billy Beer remained in production less than two years, dropping out of the public eye even before brother Jimmy left office.

Q. "I was five years old the first time I got drunk. It was on a hot day, and my father was ploughing in the field. I was sent from the house, half a mile away, to carry to him a pail of beer. . . . First I sipped the foam. I was disappointed. The preciousness evaded me. . . . I buried my face in the foam and lapped the solid liquid underneath. It wasn't good at all. But still I drank." With these words, the author describes the beginning of a life of alcoholism, which culminated in his death by suicide at age 40. The book was called *John Barleycorn— Alcoholic Memoirs,* and when it was published in 1913, it became a favorite resource of temperance lecturers and it surely gave the Prohibition movement valuable ammunition, coming as it did from one of America's most popular authors. What is his name?

A. At the time that *John Barleycorn* was published, Jack London was already famous and well on the road to wealth, as a result of his best-selling novels *The Call of the Wild,* in 1903, and *The Sea Wolf,* in 1904. London says many times in *John Barleycorn* that he didn't like the taste of beer: "I had no moral disinclination for beer, and just because I didn't like the taste of it and the weight of it was no reason I should forego the honour of his company. It was his whim to drink beer, and to have me drink beer with him. Very well, I would put up with the passing discomfort." He depicts himself as succumbing to social pressure again and again, without ever reflecting on the personal vulnerability that led him to do so. The only solution he could see was to banish alcohol altogether. He died in 1916, without ever seeing the fiasco of Prohibition.

Q. Up until the 1890s, beer bottles were sealed with corks or, even more commonly in the later years, with ceramic and/ or rubber stoppers that were wired to the bottle top. The final answer to beer bottle stopper problems, the familiar metal crown that we all know and love to this day, was patented in 1892. Who was this unsung hero, the man who invented the crown cap, to whom we all owe so much?

A. William Painter. The metal crown had a little disk of cork in it from the beginning, in order to prevent leakage. Later on, a cheaper composition cork, blended with an adhesive product, replaced the natural cork and actually improved the sealing quality of the crown. How about a toast for old Willie?

Q. Innovations often seem to stem from California, and this one is no exception. In the fall of 1982, William Boam tried to introduce a new beer into the state, but the righteous members of the state Alcoholic Beverage Control (ABC) Board denied him permission to market the beer in California, saying that it was "contrary to public welfare and morals." What was the name of the beer and what was at issue?

A. It sounded like a great idea. Boam called his brew Nude Beer, and the label featured a nude woman, visible from the waist up. He planned to change the picture each month, running nationwide contests to choose each of the young lovelies. What the ABC objected to, of course, was the label. The beer itself was to be produced via an arrangement with the Eastern Brewing Company of Hammonton, New Jersey. Nude Beer finally made it past the ABC by covering the lovelies with an opaque film, easily wiped off by the beer drinker to reveal a naked torso.

Q. Reputations are pretty fragile sometimes. Father Mohr for a while was the priest at St. Nicholas Church in Oberndorf, near Salzburg. He was a friendly fellow and often joined in with the men when they drank beer and sang off-color tavern songs. That wasn't very popular with the bishop, and Father

Mohr was removed. In Oberndorf: "It is remembered that he taught the men that if a stein or glass of beer looked like it was going to foam over as it was poured, all you had to do was to poke your finger down into the stein or glass and it would definitely not foam over. This is a very useful bit of knowledge at times and was deeply appreciated." Nobody paid much attention to the song that Father Mohr wrote with Herr Gruber, December 23, 1818. They just sort of took it for granted, unaware that it was to become one of the most popular Christmas carols of all time. What is its name?

A. For all our information about Father Mohr, we are indebted to George and Berthe Herter, who wrote the improbable but vastly interesting *Bull Cook and Authentic Historical Recipes and Practices*. Father Mohr and Herr Gruber wrote "Silent Night" as a piece for the children's chorus, to be accompanied by the composers on guitars. They did this because the church organ was on the fritz. A month later, the repairman came and fixed the organ and stole "Silent Night," later publishing it without giving any credit to the real composers. According to the Herters, "When they were old dying men, they were finally acknowledged as the true creators of "Silent Night," but were given none of the money that the song had earned. They both died as poor as church mice. . . . If you ever sing this song in your home, church, or on television, send a donation to the Father Mohr Memorial Chapel Statue Fund, Oberndorf, Austria. When they get enough, they will put up a statue of Father Mohr; he certainly deserves one. Better yet, make your donation the price of a six-pack of good beer; he would understand this."

Q. Wine drinkers are notorious for taking their beverages very seriously. Beer drinkers can be a serious lot, too, but most of us don't mind a laugh at the expense of our brew. One beer that comes out each Christmastime specializes in a particular style of offbeat humor. The label boldly proclaims: "The pale, stale ale for the pale, stale male," and it has been advertised as the only beer with the foam on the bottom. What is the brand?

A.   Olde Frothingslosh is the Pittsburgh Brewing Company's regular Iron City brew put out in a holiday costume, sometimes with an overstuffed bathing beauty featured on the can. Ivan Preston, in *The Great American Blow-Up*, tells the story of a woman customer who bought the beer to amuse friends at a party, and was very upset to find that the foam was *not* on the bottom, after all. She demanded her money back and was very upset when her wishes were denied. She went so far as to speak to a lawyer about bringing suit, but the matter died there. Some people can't take a joke.

Q.   If you are a person who favors realism when you look at paintings, you may be familiar with the works of John Sloan, an American artist who lived from 1872 to 1951. He was recognized as one of the foremost American painters of his day, but alas, it was not until he reached his seventies that he was able to support himself on the proceeds of his art work. As a struggling artist, one of Sloan's indulgences was the beer at a bar on East Seventh Street in New York. It is only fitting, then, that some of his earliest successes were with paintings of the proprietor presiding over the taps, and of customers joyfully being served mugs of the saloon's private label ale. What is the name of this still-glorious saloon?

A.   A human being can live a full life—generously, righteously, struggling always to work hard and to maintain a thoughtful mind—and in one moment of infamy, that solid reputation will be wiped out and a reputation will forever after be derived from a single, sordid act. It's that way with McSorley's Old Ale House in New York City, the subject of five Sloan paintings between 1912 and 1930. Ever since 1854, the worn sawdust-covered floor, the mug-battered bar, have hosted patrons interested in an honest drink and a comfortable atmosphere conducive to comaraderie and good conversation. Ironically, McSorley's most famous moment was on August 11, 1970, when a federal order forced McSorley's to accept female patronage. There is still only one toilet, however, and women desirous of using the stall must pass the gauntlet of men facing up to urinals amost as large as doorways.

Q.   I remember reading that Eskimos have some fifty words to describe snow and snowing, all of which suggests that as you really get to know something, you become aware of subtle but identifiable differences that might elude others. Now, how many terms do you suppose the Germans have to describe the differing types and degrees of drunkenness?

A.   According to LaVerne Rippley, author of *Of German Ways*, the answer depends on whether you speak High German or Low German, there being 111 terms for varying degrees of inebriation in the former and only 56 in the latter.

Q.   "We knew that while bock beer lasted the eltern would be gayer, kinder. We knew that while bock beer lasted, pretzels would be free at all beer saloon counters, and patrons, moved to song, would grow hoarse in saengerfests. We knew that while bock beer lasted there would be many who would marry, some even for a second time, and second weddings were twice as much fun. We knew that with bock beer and pinochle the grown-ups would let the evenings stretch and give us our fill of games and peanuts. For bock beer was the dark and ripened beverage with which the breweries of old St. Louis hailed the Risen Lord and the end of the Lenten season. All the saloons had it on Easter morning."

So says Lucille Kohler in a nostalgic short story entitled "Bock Beer Days in St. Louis." But what is bock beer?

A.   Bock beer is a strong, bottom-fermented beer, tradition-ally over 6 percent alcohol, usually dark brown in color, with a sweet malt flavor. The beer originally stemmed from Saxony in Germany, but now is produced in many places, customarily being brewed in the winter for release in the spring. Dop-pelbock is quite similar, but about double the alcohol content, usually in the 7.5 to 13 percent range.

Q.   Many different animals have graced the labels of various beers over the course of history—the bulldog, eagle, camel, rooster, giraffe, elephant, tiger, bear, etc. However, the most enduring creature on a beer label is probably the goat, which appears on many labels of bock beer. *Bock,* in German, means goat. How did the goat come to be associated with this par-ticular type of beer?

A.   There are a variety of stories about the association of bock beer with goats. The standard explanation is that the beer was first brewed in the German city of Einbeck, whose name was confused by some folks, resulting in "ein Bock," the German name for a male goat. However, the explanation I prefer comes from George and Berthe Herter: "Doctors in Einbeck, Ger-many, and the surrounding territory prescribed for people who had trouble going to sleep at night two glasses of the dark beer before bedtime to make the patient sleepy. Instead of making men sleepy, it acted as an aphrodisiac and made them chase their wives around the room. The beer was called Bock beer by the wives, meaning an oversexed male goat."

Q.   Have you ever wondered why most beer advertisements are so monotonously the same? There are a lot of songs and jingles, many celebrities lifting a glass, and lots of ordinary people reaching for a brew at the end of a hard day of work or sport. Yet you never see anyone actually drinking a beer, and there is hardly any mention of any specifics which would differentiate one beer from another. What's going on?

A. Most of our advertising guidelines are still heavily influenced by Prohibition mentality. A "voluntary" television advertisers code prohibits showing people actually drinking beer. The Federal Alcohol Administration Act prohibits "Any statement that is disparaging of a competitor's products. . . . The advertisement shall not contain any statement of alcoholic content—or any statement, design, or device representing that the use of any malt beverage has curative or therapeutic effects. . . ." There is apparently some room for discretion here, but the regulations, in effect (says George Bishop in *The Booze Reader*), permit "no references to be made which are likely to create the impression that the consumption of a malt beverage would be conducive to health and well-being. These include words and phrases such as 'bracing,' 'invigorating,' 'clears your throat,' and 'relaxes you,' when any man who has quaffed a cold beer on a warm day knows full well that it is and does all of these things." Apparently the British are every bit as muddle-headed on this subject as we are. According to Alan Wykes in *Ale and Hearty,* "Undoubtedly the most famous slogan for selling beer [in Britain] . . . was 'Guinness is good for you'—a slogan no longer permitted, some fatuous Act of Parliament having stuck its silly nose in on the ground that *no* form of alcohol is good for you and it's wicked to tell people that it is."

Q. Brewer's yeast is very big on the health food circuit. It is sold as "nature's wonder food," one of the best sources of B-complex vitamins, all the essential amino acids, and many minerals including chromium, selenium, and potassium. However, brewer's yeast has one *major* problem from a consumer's point of view. Do you know what it is?

A. The stuff tastes dreadful. Most brewer's yeast has traditionally been scraped off the top of the wort at the conclusion of fermentation, where it grows with enormous vigor, proliferating on the malt sugars as it produces alcohol. The junk accumulated in this fashion contains lots of hop oils and is extremely bitter. The brewers try to debitter the yeast and sell it to the health food companies, but with only incomplete success on both counts. The latter are increasingly selling brewer's yeast (*S. cerevisiae*) that has absolutely no connection with brewers, instead being grown on molasses or sugar beets. This product is even said to be edible and at least one company advertises that it has achieved a "superb taste." The brewers, for their part, are seeking other uses for the by-products of fermentation. Anheuser-Busch, which was the nation's largest supplier of brewer's yeast in the 1940s and 1950s, now processes the stuff and sells it as an autolyzed yeast extract, which is used as a high-protein flavor-enhancer for use in hams, sausages, soups, and crackers. If you check the ingredients label on your next can of soup or box of crackers, it may say "autolyzed yeast extract" or "natural flavoring." Now you know its origin.

Q. "Life isn't all beer and skittles; but beer and skittles, or something better of the same sort, must form a good part of every Englishman's education." That's what Thomas Hughes says in *Tom Brown's School Days*, and I kind of like the sound of it. However, not one person in a hundred knows what skittles are these days. Do you?

A. Skittles is a game that was associated with English pubs for at least a couple of centuries. Also known as ninepins, it required nine large oval-headed pins arranged in a diamond or square. The object of the game was to knock over the pins with a bowling ball (either wood or rubber, weighing 10 to 14 pounds) in as few tries as possible. The rules and scoring were highly variable, but gambling on the results was extremely common. An associated term was "to skittle away" money, referring to careless wagering.

Q. One of baseball's most colorful characters ever, the pioneer base stealer of the game, was once criticized by *Sporting News* for holding up an exhibition game, during which time he "quaffed beer with disreputable characters in the grandstand." Who was this man who dominated baseball in the 1880s?

A. Mike Kelly, otherwise known as "King Kel," was memorialized in a popular 1889 song, "Slide, Kelly, Slide." He was a great catcher, a good right fielder, and a legendary base runner. When asked by a reporter if he drank during a game, he replied, "It depends on the length of the game." When he retired from baseball in 1893, he had a brief fling on the stage and then opened up a New York saloon with a famous umpire of the day, "Honest John" Kelly. The saloon was named The Two Kels. King Kel caught pneumonia the same year and died just short of his thirty-seventh birthday.

Q. In 1777, the then German monarch wrote: "It is disgusting to notice the increase in the quantity of coffee used by my subjects. If possible, this must be prevented. My people must drink beer. His Majesty was brought up on beer and so were his ancestors, and his officers and soldiers." Who was this famous king of Prussia?

A. Frederick II (also known as "the Great") was mainly concerned that the royal treasury was being drained in order to support the new Prussian passion for the coffee bean. While Frederick was brought up on beer, his upbringing was not so happy in other respects. His father, Frederick William I, couldn't stand him, thinking him to be too frivolous and sensitive, and threw him in jail and beheaded one of his friends to toughen up young Frederick. The young prince became king at age 28, and he held the throne for forty-six years. History records that, despite his father's concerns, the man was tough enough for the job, and he ruled with a fair hand. Poor Frederick the Great, however, would be distressed to learn that coffee replaced beer as Germany's number-one beverage in the mid-1970s.

Q.   It is said that the greatest playwright of all time, William Shakespeare, improvised many of his best lines over a glass of ale at the Falcon Tavern by the Bankside in London—and at the Mermaid and the Boar's Head. No wonder ale plays such a prominent role in so many of Shakespeare's plays. How many of the following lines of the great bard can you identify?

(1) "Come on, you mad-cap. I'll to the alehouse with you presently, where, for one shot of fivepence, thou shalt have five thousand welcomes."

(2) "For a quart of ale is a dish for a king."

(3) "I would give all my fame for a pot of ale and safety."

(4) "I shall make it a felony to drink small beer."

A.   There are dozens of quotations we could have used in the question, but enough is enough. The answers are as follows: (1) *The Two Gentlemen of Verona*, Act II, Scene V. Speed is speaking to Launce. (2) *The Winter's Tale*, Act IV, Scene III. Autolycus, a relatively minor, roguish character, opens the scene by singing a song, of which the line is a part. (3) *King Henry V*, Act III, Scene II. The words are spoken by an unnamed boy, before the siege of Harfleur, surrounded by soldiers scaling ladders. (4) *King Henry VI*, Part II, Act IV, Scene II. The demagogue Jack Cade is running for office, saying that weak beer will be outlawed.

APPENDIX

CALORIC CONTENT OF BEERS BY BRAND NAME

It's not as easy to get information on calorie content of specific beers as you might think; and even when you have it, you don't know how reliable the information may be. Brewers change their recipes from time to time, and that may account for some of the discrepancies in the figures that follow. In the case of disagreement, decide for yourself which expert to trust.

Brand	Calories per 12 Ounces
Anchor Steam	154[c]
Augsberger	175[c]
Becks	150[c]
Black Horse Ale	162**
Blatz	144[c]
Brauhaus	150*
Budweiser	158*
	154**
	144[c]
Burgie!	140[a]
Busch Bavarian	158*
	146**
Carling Black Label	162*
	140**
Carlsberg Light Deluxe	153*
Carlsberg Dark 19-B	240*
Champale Malt Liquor	156*

Coors	140[c]
Country Club Malt Liquor	173*
Dos Equis	145[c]
DuBois Beer	144[a]
Falstaff	150*
Grand Union	150*
Guinness (11.4 ounces)	167[b]
Hamm's	136[c]
Heidelberg	147*
	135**
Heileman's Old Style	144[c]
Heileman's Special Export	159*
Heineken	152[c]
Henry Weinhard's Private Reserve	149[c]
Kingsbury	146*
Kirin	149[c]
Knickerbocker	160**
Kronenbourg	170[c]
Labatt's	147[c]
Löwenbräu	157[c]
Meister Brau Premium	144**
Michelob	161*
	165**
	162[c]
Miller High Life	149[c]
Molson	154[c]
North Star	165**
Old Dutch	150*
Old Milwaukee	145[c]
Old Ranger	150*
Old Style	156*
Olympia	153[c]
Pabst Blue Ribbon	150*
	152[c]
Pearl	146*
Pearl Premium	150**
Pfeifer (regular)	165**
Pfeifer (3.2)	143**

Red Cap Ale	159*
	153**
Rheingold	165*
	160**
Rolling Rock	144[c]
St. Pauli Girl	144[c]
Schaefer	159*
Schlitz	155*
	151[c]
Schmidt's	147[c]
Schmidt (3.2)	143**
Scotch Buy (Safeway)	145[c]
Stag	152*
	136**
Stroh Bohemian (regular)	150**
	149[c]
Stroh Bohemian (3.2)	136**
Tuborg	140**
	155[c]
Tudor	150*
Utica	144[a]

LIGHT BEERS

Brand	Calories per 12 Ounces
Amstel Light	96[a]
Black Label Light	96[a]
Budweiser Light	113[c]
	108[a]
Burgie! Light Golden	70[a]
Coors Light	102[c]
DuBois Ultra Light	96[a]
Erie Light	96[a]
Gablinger's Extra Light	99**
Iron City Light	96[a]
Meister Brau Lite	96**

Michelob Light	135[c]
Miller Lite	99[c]
Natural Light	110**
Olympia Gold Light	72[c]
Pabst Extra Light	68[c]
	70[a]
Pearl Light	68[a]
Red, White and Blue (Pabst)	119[a]
Schlitz Light	97[c]
	96[a]
Stag Light	96[a]
Stroh Light	116**
Utica Light	96[a]

* Netzer and Chaback: *Brand Name Calorie Counter*
** Kraus: *Calorie Guide to Brand Names and Basic Foods*
[a] CSPI: *Chemical Additives in Booze*
[b] Information obtained from the brewer
[c] *Consumer Reports*, July 1982

BIBLIOGRAPHY

The list that follows includes most of the books and several articles used in the preparation of this book. Some bits of information could not be traced to their precise source, and therefore I may have inadvertently left out a few deserving publications. I would like to comment on a few references that have been particularly useful.

No one could read much about beer and brewing without turning to Michael Jackson's thoroughly wonderful, lavishly illustrated *World Guide to Beer*. James Robertson's authoritative *Great American Beer Book* has likewise been an invaluable resource, as has the entertaining and historical account, *Brewed in America*, by Stanley Baron. I have also turned repeatedly to *The Taster's Guide to Beer* by Michael Weiner and *The Beer Book*, by Will Anderson. For a beer consumer and trivia nut, the most useful periodical is *Beer* magazine, published by McMullen Publishing, Inc.

Likewise, no one can diet—let alone write about dieting—without referring to various calorie guides. Of course, various producers and packagers of prepared foods have provided valuable information, but I would like to pay special tribute to Corinne Netzer (author of *The Brand Name Calorie Counter*); Elaine Chaback (*The Complete Calorie Counter*); and Barbara Kraus (*Calorie Guide to Brand Names and Basic Foods*).

Adams, Ramon F. *Western Words.* Norman, Oklahoma: University of Oklahoma Press, 1968.

Amis, Kingsley. *On Drink.* New York: Harcourt Brace Jovanovich, 1973.

Anderson, Will. *The Breweries of Brooklyn.* Scranton, Pennsylvania: limited edition published by the author, 1976.

Bach, Paul J., and Schaefer, James M. "The Tempo of Country Music and the Rate of Drinking in Bars." *Journal of Studies on Alcohol,* 40 (11):1058–9, 1979.

Ball, Mia. *The Worshipful Company of Brewers.* London: Hutchinson Benham, 1977.

Baring-Gould, William S. *Nero Wolfe of West Thirty-Fifth Street.* New York: Viking Press, 1969.

Barker, Dudley. *G. K. Chesterton.* Briarcliff Manor, N.Y.: Stein and Day, 1973.

Baron, Stanley. *Brewed in America—A History of Beer and Ale in the United States.* Boston: Little, Brown & Company, 1962.

Batchelor, Denzil. *The English Inn.* London: B. T. Batsford Ltd., 1963.

Beer and America Since Repeal. East Stroudsburg, Pennsylvania: Modern Brewery, Inc., 1936.

Behan, Brendan. *Borstal Boy.* New York: Alfred A. Knopf, 1959.

Berland, Theodore. *Consumer Guide Rating the Diets.* New York: New American Library, 1980.

Bickerdyke, John. *The Curiosities of Ale and Beer.* London: Spring Books, originally published 1889 (facsimile 1965).

Birmingham, Frederic. *Falstaff's Complete Beer Book.* New York: Universal Award House, 1970.

Bishop, George. *The Booze Reader.* Los Angeles: Sherbourne Press, 1965.

Bohren, Craig F., and Brown, Gail M. "Cloud Physics in a Glass of Beer." *Weatherwise,* 34(5):221–4, October 1981.

Brown, J.F. *Guinness and Hops.* London: Arthur Guinness & Son, 1980.

Brown, Sanborn C. *Wines and Beers of Old New England.* Hanover, New Hampshire: University Press of New England, 1978.

Carter, Hugh Alton. *Cousin Beedie and Cousin Hot.* Englewood Cliffs, New Jersey: Prentice-Hall, 1978.

Chaback, Elaine. *The Complete Calorie Counter.* New York: Dell Publishing, 1979.

Connery, Donald S. *The Scandinavians.* New York: Simon & Schuster, 1966.

Creamer, Robert W. *Babe—The Legend Comes to Life.* New York: Simon & Schuster, 1974.

Cruso, Thalassa. *To Everything There Is a Season.* New York: Alfred A. Knopf, 1973.

Cutright, Paul Russell. *Theodore Roosevelt—The Naturalist.* New York: Harper & Brothers, 1956.

Della Femina, Jerry. *From Those Wonderful Folks Who Gave You Pearl Harbor.* New York: Simon & Schuster, 1970.

Denison, Merrill. *The Barley and the Stream—The Molson Story.* Toronto: McClelland & Stewart Ltd., 1955.

Despain, R.O. *The Malt-Ease Flagon.* Berkeley: Ten Speed Press, 1978.

Diamant, Lincoln. *Television's Classic Commercials.* New York: Hastings House, 1971.

Dickey, James. *Deliverance.* Boston: Houghton Mifflin, 1970.

Donaldson, Gerald and Lampert, Gerald (eds.). *The Great Canadian Beer Book.* Toronto: McClelland & Stewart Ltd., 1975.

Downard, William. *The Cincinnati Brewing Industry.* Athens, Ohio: University Press, 1973.

Durso, Joseph. *The All-American Dollar—The Big Business of Sports.* Boston: Houghton Mifflin Company, 1971.

Erbe, Ron. *The American Premium Guide to Baseball Cards.* Florence, Ala.: Americana, 1982.

Fisher, M.F.K. *The Art of Eating.* New York: Vintage Books, 1976.

Fleischer, Nat. *John L. Sullivan.* New York: G.P. Putnam's Sons, 1951.

Fleming, Ian. *Thrilling Cities.* New York: New American Library, 1964.

Flexner, Stuart Berg. *I Hear America Talking.* New York: Van Nostrand Reinhold Company, 1976.

Forbis, William H. (ed.) *John Gunther's Inside Australia.* New York: Harper & Row, 1972.

Fowler, Gene. *Good Night, Sweet Prince—The Life and Times of John Barrymore.* Philadelphia: The Blakiston Company, 1943.

Clifford Gastineau et al. (ed.) *Fermented Food—Beverages in Nutrition.* New York: Academic Press, 1979.

Getlein, Frank and Dorothy. *The Bite of the Print.* New York: Clarkson Potter, Inc., 1963.

Glyn, Anthony. *The Blood of a Britishman.* Newton Abbott: Readers Union, 1971.

Gollin, James. *Worldly Goods.* New York: Random House, 1971.

Gunther, John. *Twelve Cities.* New York: Harper and Row, 1967.

Hacker, Andrew. *U/S—A Statistical Portrait of the American People.* New York: Viking, 1983.

Hackwood, Frederick. *Inns, Ales and Drinking Customs of Old New England.* New York: Sturgis and Walton Company, circa 1909.

Halsey, William F. *Admiral Halsey's Story.* New York: McGraw-Hill, 1947.

Haetron, Philip G. *The Intellectual Life.* London: MacMillan and Company, 1890.

Hardwick, W.A., et al. "N-Nitrosodimethylamine in Malt Beverages—Anticipatory Action by the Brewing Industry." *Regulatory Toxicology and Pharmacology.* 2:38–66, 1982.

Harris, Nathaniel. *The Art of Manet.* New York: Excalibur Books, 1982.

Hassall, Christopher. *Ambrosia and Small Beer.* New York: Harcourt Brace and World, 1965.

Held, John, Jr. *My Pious Friends and Drunken Companions.* New York: The Macauley Company, 1927.

Herter, George Leonard, and Herter, Berthe. *Bull Cook and Authentic Historical Recipes and Practices.* Waseca, Minnesota: Herters, Inc., 1971.

Hoagland, Edward. *African Calliope—A Journey to the Sudan.* New York: Random House, 1979.

Hough, Donald. *The Cocktail Hour in Jackson Hole.* New York: W.W. Norton, 1956.

Houston, Alice W. *The American Heritage Book of Fish Cookery.* New York: American Heritage Publishing Company, 1980.

Hunt, Peter (comp.). *Eating & Drinking—An Anthology for Epicures.* London: Ebury Press, 1961.

Hunter, Beatrice Trum. *Fermented Foods and Beverages.* New Canaan, Conn.: Keats Publishing, 1973.

Ives, Burl. *Wayfaring Stranger.* New York: Whittlesey House, 1948.

Johns, Bud. *The Ombibulous Mr. Mencken.* San Francisco: Synergistic Press, 1968.

Johnson, William Weber. *Kelly Blue.* New York: Doubleday and Co., 1960.

Kaplan, Frederick, and Keijzer, Arne de. *The China Guidebook.* Boston: Houghton Mifflin, 1982.

Kennedy, Diana. *The Cuisines of Mexico.* New York: Harper and Row, 1972.

Kerouac, Jack. *On the Road.* New York: Viking, 1957.

King, Frank A. *Beer Has a History.* London: Hutchinson's Scientific and Technical Publications, 1947.

Kouwenhoven, John A. *The Beer Can by the Highway.* New York: Doubleday, 1961.

Kraus, Barbara. *Calorie Guide to Brand Names and Basic Foods.* New York: New American Library, 1982.

Kress, Roland. *Making Friends Is Our Business—100 Years of Anheuser-Busch.* St. Louis: Anheuser-Busch, Inc., 1953.

Kronenberger, Louis (ed.). *The Best Plays of 1957–1958.* New York: Dodd Mead and Company, 1968.

Lawson, Donna. *Mother Nature's Beauty Cupboard.* London: Robert Hale & Company, 1973.

Lee, Kay, and Lee, Marshall. *The Illuminated Book of Days.* New York: G.P. Putnam, 1979.

Lender, Mark E., and Martin, James K. *Drinking in America— A History.* New York: The Free Press, 1982.

Lipske, Michael, et al. *Chemical Additives in Booze.* Washington, D.C.: Center for Science in the Public Interest, 1982.

London, Jack. *John Barleycorn or Alcoholic Memoirs.* Cambridge, Massachusetts: Robert Bentley, Inc., 1964.

Martells, Jack. *The Beer Can Collectors Bible.* New York: Ballantine Books, 1976.

Martin, Robert Bernard. *Tennyson—The Unquiet Heart.* Oxford, England: Clarendon Press, 1980.

Maugham, Somerset. *Cakes and Ale (and Twelve Short Stories).* New York: Doubleday and Company, 1967.

Mercatante, Anthony S. *Who's Who in Egyptian Mythology.* New York: Clarkson Potter Inc., 1978.

Millard, Arnold A. *History of the Carson Brewing Company.* Carson City, Nev.: The Brewery Press, 1980.

Morris, William and Mary. *Dictionary of Word and Phrase Origins,* vol. 2. New York: Harper and Row, 1967.

Muir, Frank. *An Irreverent and Thoroughly Incomplete Social History of Almost Everything.* Briarcliff Manor, N.Y.: Stein and Day, 1976.

Netzer, Corinne (with Elaine Chaback). *The Brand-Name Calorie Counter.* New York: Dell Publishing Co., 1978.

Ogilvy, David. *Blood, Brains and Beer.* New York: Atheneum, 1978.

Ojala, Reino. *Twenty Years of American Beers—the 30's and 40's.* Minnesota: published by the author, date unknown.

Osborne, Keith, and Pipe, Brian. *The International Book of Beer Labels, Mats, and Coasters.* Middlesex, England: Hamlyn Publishing Group Limited, 1979.

Pepe, Phil, and Hollander, Zander. *The Book of Sports Lists # 3.* New York: Pinnacle Books, 1981.

Porter, William H. (O. Henry) *The Complete Works of O. Henry.* New York: Doubleday and Co., 1953.

Pozen, Morris A. *Successful Brewing.* Chicago: Brewery Age Publishing Company, 1935.

Price, Lorna. *The Plan of St. Gall in Brief.* Berkeley, California: University of California Press, 1982.

Raban, Jonathan. *Old Glory—An American Voyage.* New York: Simon & Schuster, 1981.

Rapport, Samuel, and Schartle, Patricia. *America Remembers.* New York: Hanover House, 1956.

Reid, Jan. *The Improbable Rise of Redneck Rock.* New York: DaCapo Press/Plenum, 1977.

Reid, J.C. (ed.) *A Book of New Zealand.* Glasgow: Collins, 1964.

Ringo, Miriam. *Nobody Said It Better!* Chicago: Rand McNally and Company, 1980.

Rippley, LaVern. *Of German Ways.* Minneapolis, Minn.: Dillon Press, 1979.

Ritchie, Donald. *The Inland Sea.* New York: Weatherhill, 1971.

Robertson, James D. *The Great American Beer Book.* New York: Warner Books, 1978.

Rosenthal, Eric. *Tankards and Tradition.* Cape Town: Howard Timmins, 1961.

Royko, Mike. *Boss.* New York: E.P. Dutton and Company, 1971.

Smith, H. Allen. *The Life and Legend of Gene Fowler.* New York: William Morrow and Company, 1977.

———. *The Pig in the Barber Shop.* Boston: Little, Brown and Company, 1958.

Smith, Willie the Lion. *Music on My Mind.* New York: Doubleday and Company, 1964.

Steinbeck, John. *East of Eden.* New York: Viking Press, 1952.

———. *Sweet Thursday.* New York: Viking Press, 1954.

———. *The Log from the Sea of Cortez.* New York: Viking Press, 1941.

Steiner's Guide to American Hops. S. S. Steiner, Inc., 1973.

Stewart, Larry. "Beer—The Drink of Choice Among Runners." *Runners World,* March 1981.

Stunkard, Albert J. (ed.) *Obesity.* Philadelphia: W.B. Saunders, 1980.

Schickele, Peter. *The Definitive Biography of P.D.Q. Bach.* New York: Random House, 1976.

Scott, Jack Denton. *Passport to Adventure.* New York: Random House, 1966.

Seranne, Ann, and Tebbel, John (eds.). *The Epicure's Companion.* New York: David McKay, 1962.

Seward, Jack. *The Japanese.* New York: William Morrow and Company, 1972.

Shapiro, Nat (ed.). *Popular Music,* vol. 4. New York: Adrian Press, 1968.

Tannahill, Reay. *Food in History.* Briarcliff Manor, N.Y.: Stein and Day, 1973.

Theroux, Paul, *The Great Railway Bazaar.* Boston: Houghton Mifflin, 1975.

———. *The Old Patagonian Express.* Boston: Houghton Mifflin, 1979.

Thomas, Dylan. *Adventures in the Skin Trade.* New York: New Directions Books, 1955.

Thompson, Toby. *Saloon.* New York: Grossman Publishers, 1976.

Tolbert, Frank X. *A Bowl of Red.* New York: Doubleday and Company, 1972.

Trager, James. *The Food Book.* New York: Flare Books, 1970.

Trillin, Calvin. *Alice, Let's Eat.* New York: Random House, 1978.

Tyler, Anne. *Dinner at the Homesick Restaurant.* New York: A.A. Knopf, 1982.

Villas, James. *American Taste.* New York: Arbor House, 1982.

Watney, John. *Beer Is Best.* London: Peter Owen Publishing, 1974.

Weiner, Michael. *The Taster's Guide to Beer.* New York: Collier Books, 1977.

Wolfe, Tom. *The Right Stuff.* New York: Farrar Straus Giroux, 1979.

Wren, Christopher S. *Winners Got Scars Too—The Life and Legends of Johnny Cash.* New York: Dial Press, 1971.

Wright, William Aldis (ed.). *The Complete Works of William Shakespeare.* New York: Garden City Books, 1936.

Wykes, Alan. *Ale and Hearty.* London: Jupiter Books, 1979.

IMPORTANT NOTICE

Do you know a bit of beer trivia that somehow escaped being included in this book? Some bit of information, a story, a quotation, or anything that ties beer in with the rest of the world in which we live? If so, send it to me at the address below. If this book is successful enough to warrant a sequel, and I am able to use your information, you will be given full credit in print—and you will be sent a complimentary copy of the book in which your item appears.

Send all beer trivia (with some information about where you found it, so I can check for accuracy when appropriate) to: Martin Lipp, M.D., P.O. Box 26393, San Francisco, CA 94126.

INDEX

ABOUT THE AUTHOR

Martin Lipp has been a physician almost twenty years, and he has been dieting and drinking beer even longer than that. His credentials for writing this book are appropriately stuffy: he is an associate professor on a medical school faculty, he has published numerous papers in scientific journals, and he is the author of two previous books, including an extremely well-received handbook for physicians on the doctor-patient relationship called *Respectful Treatment—The Human Side of Medical Care*. His medical practice is restricted to emergency medicine (real blood-and-guts stuff), and his social life tends to focus on good food and good friends accompanied by good brew and occasionally wine. Dr. Lipp knows about diets: he has a collection of 250 diet books in his own library and customarily loses the same ten to fifteen pounds several times a year.